Communicating Midwifery

Twenty years of experience

Caroline Flint

SRN, SCM, ADM

with sections introduced by Deborah Hughes

Books for Midwives Press
Books for Midwives Press is a joint publishing collaboration
between The Royal College of Midwives and
Haigh and Hochland Publications Ltd

Published by Books for Midwives Press, 174a Ashley Road, Hale, Cheshire, WA15 9SF, England

© 1995, Caroline Flint

First edition

ISBN 1-898507-19-8

British Library Cataloguing in Publication Data
A catalogue record for this book is available from the British Library

Printed in Great Britain by Cromwell Press Ltd

Contents

Introduction

When I was eight my mother had her fourth child at home. I can remember my sister as if it were yesterday. A small red soft sweetly-smelling baby, the soft down of her black hair, the little snuffling noises. I thought she was utterly, utterly, magical and at that moment I resolved that I would become a midwife and that if I could, I would have lots of babies.

I have been fortunate to have achieved both these ambitions in my life. I have given birth to three beautiful and talented children (a totally unbiased view of course!) and I have found the most enormous fulfilment in my life and work as a midwife.

My mother has been a significant influence on my life. She hated midwives, the stories she told of the midwives who had looked after her during her six pregnancies were of bossy, domineering women, who were unkind to their suffering patients, without sensitivity, without sympathy, and without feelings. At the birth of my sister at home she asked the GP if he would come because she knew he was kind and although he didn't deliver the baby he was there to give her support. My father was not at any of our births. At my birth he was off fighting in the war and for the births of my siblings he would not have been allowed in to the Labour Ward, because in those days men were kept out – it was women's business.

When I became pregnant with my first baby I decided to have him at home because men were still kept out of the delivery rooms and I knew I couldn't go through the obviously painful process without Giles to hold my hand and support me. I also felt that I would not naturally be a very good mother and knowing that I'm brilliant at delegating I was afraid that if I was in hospital I would delegate my baby to whoever happened to be passing rather than look after it myself. I knew that for me to become a mother it was important that I had my baby at home and to be totally responsible for the baby. I also hate not being in control of my environment and I knew that in hospital it would be more difficult for me, whereas at home the midwife would be the visitor to my flat.

For both Giles and me the birth of our first child Matthew was a magical experience. We had the most loving, kind and enthusiastic midwife, Sister Harrap. Despite the slight handicap (in the days of pinard stethoscopes) of being deaf and therefore being unable to listen to the fetal heart, and despite not doing vaginal examinations because she said that you could look at a woman and see from her outward demeanour how far on in labour she was, I found her loving care of me incredibly supportive and it helped to make the birth of my first son the most empowering experience of my life, for which I shall always be grateful to such a beautiful and loving midwife.

Before Matthew's birth, and then again during my next two pregnancies I went to NCT classes. For me they were a very profound educational experience. They were one of the first of the women's groups, my first brush with feminism, a place where ones feeling were acknowledged as being important, not just some emotional rubbish. The NCT was a revelation to me.

After the birth of my next two children, Rebecca and Thomas, I started to teach for the National Childbirth Trust and have continued to do so ever since. Every week couples sit in my sitting-room and tell me about the momentous experience they are approaching and what they feel about it and what they feel about the care they are receiving from the NHS. The reason that I am so passionately committed to continuity of carer for women is that week after week in my sitting-room women have said to me 'if only we knew who the midwife was going to be, if only we could get to know her'. I have been educated by women who have shared with me their feelings, their fears and their thoughts and by men who have guided me, helped me not to be sexist and enlightened me as to how they want to support their partners.

These then are two of the influences on my life but probably the strongest influence on my life has been Giles, my husband. He is a lawyer, committed to justice, equity and totally opposed to discrimination for racial or religious reasons and very much committed to equality of the sexes. I have learnt so much from his wise and patient (and sometimes impatient!) counsel. He has been able to advise my friends when they have been in trouble and he has advised me when I have been having problems. Those same friends that I have made throughout my professional career, many of whom are members of the Association of Radical Midwives, have also been a great influence on my thinking and behaviour. Most of my friends (and I) have been in trouble within the midwives' rather punitive disciplinary system. It has been so good and so strengthening to have their support when times have been hard, so useful to have their ideas and thoughts. Often I think that it is not me who is the thinker, it's just that I seem to be able to put other people's thoughts into words on paper.

I don't know why I have written so many articles – it may just be that I am an opinionated woman but I do know that if I don't get things off my chest by writing them down I nearly burst. It's also one of the most effective ways I know of achieving change. If I write something down – even if it is only a thought, then I know someone will read it and they may be interested in the idea or it may trigger a response in them. Then if someone asks me to speak about what I have written I can elaborate and share ideas with other people who will elaborate on the idea and improve it. My great fortune in having visited Australia seven times, New Zealand twice, Malta, Iceland, Guernsey, Holland, Norway, Denmark and several other lovely places is all because I have written articles and had them published in some of the journals. I do urge every midwife to follow suit. If I can write so can you. I only write in the same way that I write letters to my Mum – you could do this as well.

I know that I could not have written so much without the support of Giles, who often patiently cooks a meal or does what has to be done while I sit glued to the word processor pouring out the things that I hold in my heart that I can't rest until I have got down on paper. Nowadays the process of writing is much easier for me because my dear friend, Janet Andrews, who also works as a secretary and administrator for our Practice, types out my articles which I have dictated into a dictating machine. The support that I have received from Giles, Janet and the children and my colleagues, Valerie Taylor and Hiromi Takahashi, has enabled me to produce these articles over the years. I hope you will find them of interest. For me it is humbling and sometimes frustrating to read words I wrote ten or fifteen years ago and to realize that the changes that I was hoping for then haven't yet come to pass, but maybe they will soon, who knows?

As President of the Royal College of Midwives I hope that it will be easier to achieve some of the objectives I have held for many years. It is a large and very exciting organization and the staff at the RCM are devoted and extremely hard working. Members and Council members are extremely committed both to midwifery and to women. All are determined to improve the services available during pregnancy and childbirth and many, many of us hold the same vision – perhaps the time is ripe now?

I would like to thank Deb Hughes for the introductions that she has written to every group of articles. She has made me laugh and brought back many memories of our long and much appreciated friendship. I would also like to thank Henry Hochland for producing this book and for all the work he does for midwives and, through them, for women.

Caroline Flint
May 1995.

Midwives, not Nurses

It is doubtless ironic that all the articles in this section originally appeared in *Nursing Times*. Caroline was a contributor to their weekly opinion column 'Arena' from its inauguration in 1984 until 1987. She was also, during the same period, *Nursing Times* midwifery associate editor. Four of the articles were written for 'Arena' and are primarily journalistic pieces aiming to raise controversial or topical issues in a provocative way. It was, however, the fifth and more finished article, which predated 'Arena' that ruffled most feathers; midwives' knickers being seen by many at that time to be a subject which brought the profession into disrepute. It seemed that if midwives aspiring to professional status had bottoms, it certainly wasn't the thing to do to draw attention to the fact. The unfortunate tendency for most midwifery uniforms to do just that was, of course, the point of the article. More than a decade later, midwives' behinds may not be on the agenda but they are still on show or accentuated by the uniforms worn in most units.

The theme of the section is the real or desired independence of midwifery from nursing: historical, political and philosophical. (Political independence is considered at greater length in Section Four). Two of the articles look at uniform, one looks at the aspirations of the Royal College of Nurses in relation to midwives, one questions the desirability of pursuing a nursing qualification prior to entering midwifery and the other describes three positive events in midwifery in 1985, all of which have been developed with some degree of success during the intervening decade.

The uniform issue, as already mentioned, rumbles on. A few units have abandoned them altogether, whilst a few more have taken 'the sweatshirt approach', combining a corporate image (the sweatshirt) with 'mufti' below the waist. Caroline herself has been working independently since 1986, thus liberating herself from her 'skimpy skirt' (see 'Symbols of Servility'). Perhaps if she had continued to work in the NHS and squeeze herself into a uniform, the resulting fall-out (sic) would have meant that British midwives would have abandoned uniforms long ago. Meanwhile, under the onslaught of the changes of recent years, it seems this is an issue that is sleeping rather than dead.

Hats, on the other hand, have largely been withdrawn and seem to have disappeared from Caroline's life sometime during the period in which the articles comprising this section were written (see 'Mistaken Identity'). The hats described in 'Symbols of Servility' are those of my own Alma Mater, St George's. Caroline, coming from Guy's, does not quite seem to have grasped the full symbolic meaning of these hats. They were meant to have four pleats to symbolize the four Cardinal Virtues and 'the requisite number of ruffles' at the back was in fact three: to denote the Trinity. My own version, held together with paper clips for the most part, were probably heretical as well as grubby.

Caroline has been active in the Royal College of Midwives at both branch and national levels since 1977 and 1983 respectively. This commitment derives from the belief, shared by many, that it is the RCM which is best placed to represent midwives and lobby for improved maternity services in the UK. Others feel that the RCM is beyond redemption and that few returns are to be gained from expending energy within it. Midwives are similarly divided over the merits or otherwise of the United Kingdom Central Council for Nursing, Midwifery and Health Visiting. In 'No Surrender' Caroline shares the frustrations of many midwives with both bodies: midwives have been annexed and milked dry under current professional legislation whilst the RCM, with the exception of its Employment Affairs Department, has often seemed to lack energy and leadership. Not being one simply to criticize from the sidelines, Caroline successfully stood for election to the Presidency of the RCM in 1994. Meanwhile the Royal College of Nursing has established its Midwifery Society and some midwives (allegedly some 4000) have even joined it. It remains to be seen whether President Flint, in her opening address to a RCM annual conference will call for the annexation of the RCN Midwifery Society and provoke an outcry in the opinion columns of *Nursing Times* from irate RCN members, thereby turning this particular wheel full-circle.

Pre-registration midwifery education, previously known as 'direct entry training' (see 'Should Midwives Train as Florists?') is now well established in the United Kingdom. Yet in 1986, just nine years ago, there was only one midwifery school left offering such a course. The Association of Radical Midwives, many of whose founding members were direct entrants, had long called for an expansion of DE courses. The RCM had been less enthusiastic and a conference motion calling for such expansion failed to attract enough support to be even debated in both 1983 and 1985. For once, midwifery was helped by nursing: in 1986 the UKCC published its 'Project 2000' proposals which would have made midwifery a 'branch' of nursing and the midwifery profession united behind a earlier proposal of the English National Board to expand DE midwifery education. The actual withdrawal from 'Project 2000' was not attained however without a considerable expenditure of energy on the part of many midwives. 'No Surrender', written shortly before the 'Project 2000' report was finally published and was one of the many articles printed at that time which eventually led to the passing of a motion in support of DE courses at the RCM annual conference in July 1986 and the eventual withdrawal of midwifery from 'Project 2000'. Midwifery unity won the day.

Caroline's writing style is a constant source of both admiration and irritation. It is certainly not the detached academic style favoured by most editors and which has rendered the professional press, with the exception of ARM's 'Midwifery Matters', rather tediously uniform in style if not in content. She is frequently facetious, as she herself admits in 'No Surrender'. Her primary aim is to get her message across and she often resorts to overstatement or simplification to make a point. Examples include the rather bleak description of nurse-midwifery in 'No Surrender' which would annoy the mildest of American Certified Nurse Midwives, and the description of childbirth in 'Should Midwives Train as Florists?' as 'a normal physiological process, like having your bowels open, or breathing or making love'. She wants the reader to say 'yes' even if the affirmative is immediately followed by a 'but'.

Whatever her theme Caroline always relates the issue to clinical practice. Care should be personal and evaluated ('Mistaken Identity'), women should be supported in active birth ('No Surrender') and upright birthing positions encouraged ('Three Steps Forward', 'Should Midwives Train as Florists?'). Her belief in the right and ability of most women to give birth without intervention with the support of a known and trusted midwife is a thread which runs through this as through all other sections of this book.

Mistaken Identity

What do hotel chambermaids in Oban have in common with community midwives? Caroline Flint discovered their unusual connection during a trip to Scotland

While I was on holiday in Scotland I met a community midwife in an hotel in Oban. 'Hello', I said, going up the stairs, 'I'm Caroline Flint, midwifery associate editor of *Nursing Times.*' I held out my hand and she shook it, rather quizzically I thought, and then she said in an attractive Scots burr, 'How do you do Mrs Flint. I hope you have a lovely holiday', and bustled off. No discussion on the state of midwifery in Scotland, no little confidences - 'I've got 15 postnatals to see today, must dash'. Nothing.

I thought this was strange and I wondered who was needing midwifery care in this hotel. The average age of the residents seemed to be about 90, but then there was always the staff. I carried on up the stairs.

When I came to our floor I turned along the corridor and - lo and behold - another community midwife. The mystery was solved; these must be district nurses giving care to some of the elderly residents of the hotel. I greeted the district nurse by asking her if she had many patients here. She looked at me even more quizzically. 'I'm one of the chambermaids Madam,' she said. 'Is there any way I can help you?'

Abashed and embarrassed I asked her, 'Where do you get your uniforms from? You all look like community midwives.' 'Och' (yes Scots people really *do* say it) 'people have said that before, we get our uniforms from Alexanders, the uniform shop in town.'

Many of us have discarded our caps now that everyone from the waitresses in motorway cafés to the female assistants in the bakery department at Tesco were wearing nurses' caps, but the chambermaids of Oban really got me thinking about what we wear.

What I wear also came under discussion a few days ago when I was discussing a woman whose baby I delivered at home before the holiday. 'Tell me Juliet', I said. 'Was there anything that I did that you weren't expecting or anything that I should have warned you about beforehand?'. In other words we were having an evaluation of my treatment towards her during labour.

'I wasn't expecting your delivery clothes', she said. It turned out that towards the end of the first stage of labour I had said, 'I'm going to change into my delivery clothes now', and I had gone into the next room to put on a clean T-shirt and dark track suit trousers, and a clean pair of socks.

It turned out that she had expected a surgical cap and gown so that I would be looking as if I was about to do open heart surgery. We had a giggle about this, but it did make me think about uniform and the importance of what we wear.

The Royal College of Nursing is determined to make us all feel that we are 'nurses'. Would they even feel remotely interested in annexing midwives if we hadn't made the mistake of wearing the same clothes as nurses?

While I was in Scotland I drove past a hospital and someone in a white top came out and got into her car. 'Is she a nurse?' asked my husband. 'No, she's a physiotherapist', I answered. I knew because of what she was wearing - something which was distinctive to her profession. As she had trousers on it was also functional for the job that she has to do.

Are nurses' uniforms functional for midwives? Are the skimpy skirts really conducive to ease of movement when helping a woman who is squatting or on all fours? When we demonstrate the way a baby comes out, does the assembled audience really want glimpses of intimate parts of the midwife which no-one but her nearest and dearest should be privy to?

The freedom of wearing your own clothes is incredibly important in maintaining professional responsibility. You are responsible for ensuring that they are clean, decent and functional and that they look smart. Surely it is much better for midwives to wear their own clothes - and if we need a cover perhaps we could wear an overall?

A white coat perhaps? If this worries the medical secretaries, specimen porters, greengrocers and doctors who all claim the white coat as their own, how about a blue coat or a red coat, or a tabard?

A friend suggested that if we wear our own clothes we could be putting a barrier between us and the women we care for. If we wear really good clothes (on our salaries!) we would create a barrier between ourselves and poor women. At the moment we look so messy and awful that we make everyone feel at home. Perhaps my T-shirt and tracksuit bottoms are the answer. For most of my work I wear a tracksuit/ leisure suit/ jogging suit and there is one I have that is in the midwives' stewart blue - perhaps we could all wear them? They are certainly more practical than the silly dresses we are saddled with at the moment which have the added disadvantage that we are mistaken for another profession.

Whatever we decide upon, as a member of an old and fine profession I want to look smart, I want to wear clothes that are hygienic and functional and I don't want to be confused with a chambermaid in Oban, even though she was very friendly and she did give me an extra sachet of shampoo. I don't want to be confused with nurses either, although I admire and acknowledge their work and struggles. I belong to a profession which has an identity of its own - it's time we showed that in what we wear.

Reproduced with kind permission from Nursing Times, August 5, Vol 83, No 31, 1987

No Surrender

Midwives must resist attempts by the Royal College of Nursing to take them over, says Caroline Flint. The experience of other countries suggests that when this happens, midwives end up doing what the doctors order

So the president and general secretary of the Royal College of Nursing want to take over the midwives. This is seen in the RCN's appointment of a midwifery advisor and president Maude Storey's comments at the annual congress, when she expressed the desire to bring all branches of nursing together, including midwifery.[1]

I'm waiting next to hear the president of the Royal College of Physicians stand up and say that he wants to take over the Royal College of Surgeons. For, as he could rightly say, 'we have more in common than divides us', or the president of the Federation of Master Builders wanting to take over the Institute of Civil Engineers. Perhaps we could leave it all to the RCN. Tomorrow the midwives, the day after the doctors, next week – the world! What is happening inside the RCN that it has this power to lust to control other professions? Is its house so perfectly in order that it is being kindly to us and is going to help us along in the same way that it is helping the psychiatric nurses, the district nurses and the enrolled nurses?

I'm being facetious, but what is this fatal fascination that midwives have for other professions? The obstetricians have been busily annexing midwives for the past half century; the Central Midwives Board was peopled mainly by doctors because they wanted to have control of the midwifery profession, and insisted when the 1902 Midwives Act went through Parliament that they had more than adequate representation on the body. The trades unions have been trying to lure midwives into their ranks for

years – I shouldn't be surprised to open my newspaper tomorrow and discover that the National Union of Punch and Judy Operators want us to join their ranks.

Perhaps we should take a few tips from dentists. No-one seems to want to annex them, and it appears to me that they are in a similar position to midwives. They have similarities with another and larger profession but are very much a separate and distinct profession in their own right, with different philosophies and objectives. Perhaps it's what dentists represent that makes them secure against takeover. Perhaps midwives are so attractive because of what they do. Everyone is fascinated and entranced by young babies. The whole process of pregnancy and birth is so amazing, perhaps we who are involved in it are as irresistible as the process we are there to aid.

Which leads on to our raison d'etre – women and mothers and babies. Would they be helped if we became part of the Royal College of Nursing? Would women fare better than they do now? Would they receive more helpful and more supportive care in their role as mothers? Would nurse/midwives do it better? We don't have to look far. Nurses have annexed midwives in many countries of the world, and in many countries of the world they are called just that – nurse/midwives. They wear nurses' clothes, they do what the doctor orders, they ensure that women are quiet and given adequate sedation and that when their labour is slower than is cost-effective their labour is speeded up. They ensure that women use the nice, efficient, expensive machines which can save the messy business of putting a hand or an ear on a sweaty tum, they make sure that the environment is clean and efficient and that babies are kept clean and organized, that the woman and her baby are 'cared for'. This is a far cry from the sweaty, throaty-sounding, agonising but exultant business which I see as labour, a far cry from women taking responsibility for themselves and their health and their own babies supported by the midwives those 'with women'.

Midwives have already given a great deal to nurses. With the annexation of midwives in the Nurses, Midwives and Health Visitors Act, we have given a lead to the other professions in our code of professional conduct, our list of competencies, our statutory refresher courses and our education based on clinical practice. It would seem to me to be silly to shoot the goose laying golden eggs. If the midwives are annexed – or lured, or beguiled – into the Royal College of Nursing, where would all the ideas to copy come from?

This opening salvo does mean one thing though: the Royal College of Midwives must show the world a more public face. It needs to increase its public relations. This shouldn't be difficult. It is already doing sterling work for midwives with the Pay Review Body and in industrial relations, representing midwives in trouble. It has raised the awareness of midwives on professional issues and formulated policies for the future of midwifery and childbirth, as well as showing leadership in the formulation of educational policies. Now it needs to show dynamic leadership and an alliance with both mothers and other midwives with a more radical approach.

It is capable of doing this. But I must stop now – I've got the National Association of Dog Walkers on the phone. They want us too!

Reference

1. Storey, M. Opening address of RCN president, to the RCN Annual Congress. Glasgow, April 6, 1987.

Reproduced with kind permission from Nursing Times, May 6, Vol 83, No 18, 1987

Should Midwives Train as Florists?

This suggestion, says Caroline Flint, is only slightly more absurd than asking midwives to train as nurses before they can train to be midwives. She argues that nurse training is not only unnecessary, it can be positively harmful

Just imagine that you want to be a solicitor. You go along to your local solicitors' practice and say, 'I would like to become a solicitor', and the answer is, 'You can't become a solicitor until you have first trained as a policeman.'

'A policeman? But I don't want to be a policeman. I want to be a solicitor.'

'It's very useful for you to be a policeman first - you learn about the criminal mind, you learn a lot of basics of the law, you learn about court procedure, you learn how law affects ordinary people. You need to have been a policeman first before you become a solicitor; you learn so many useful and basic things for your future role.'

Or perhaps you feel like becoming a dentist?

'I'm sorry but before you train to be a dentist you have to do a medical training first. You must first train to be a doctor - so much of what a doctor learns in his training is enormously useful to a dentist.

Or perhaps you want to be midwife?

'Well, before you train to be a midwife you have to train to be a nurse. It will be enormously useful to you. As a nurse you will learn to take care of bedsores and to prevent them, you will be able to scrub in theatre for amputations, you will be able to look after diabetics and you will understand the signs and problems of diabetes. You will learn about congestive cardiac failure, how to make a bed, the care of people with coronary thrombosis, subarachnoid haemorrhage, concussion, how to give an injection, kidney dialysis, giving medicines - all thoroughly useful knowledge which no sane person could do without before becoming a midwife?'

Or is it?

Is it as nonsensical and wasteful as training a solicitor to be a policeman first? Or a dentist to be a doctor first? Would it be better if midwives trained to be chiropodists first? That would help them to learn how to communicate with patients, after all. Or perhaps we ought to train first as florists? We would have much prettier flower arrange–ments in the postnatal wards then.

But surely, you will say, it is really useful for a midwife to have a basic nurse training before she embarks on her midwifery training? It isn't as if she has to unlearn any of the things she has learned as a nurse, is it?

But, I would reply, what about her attitude to patients? Midwives don't have patients - they are *with women* as they go through a huge and life-changing experience. They are partners and colleagues. They work as a team, but a team of equal decision-makers. The woman is not ill, she is going through a normal physiological process, like having your bowels open, or breathing, or making love.

Perhaps a midwife needs a different attitude to the women she is with from the nurse with her patients? When you are nursing patients, they are ill. Women going through childbirth are not ill.

What about the midwife's attitude to doctors? Does that need to be in any way different to the attitude of the nurse? Surely the doctor and midwife are there for the same thing? Working as a team of professionals. Well, yes and no. Not for nothing does the midwife call herself the 'guardian of normal childbirth'. And as childbirth becomes increasingly technological, and more and more new tests and sophisticated diagnostic tools are used, a growing number of women have Caesarean sections or have their labour accelerated. It is the midwife who has the skill and knowledge to protect women from over-medicalization. She can protect them from the over-enthusiastic use of tools which might help one woman enormously, but which might be inappropriate for another woman, and may indeed interfere with the normal physiological progress of labour.

What about the attitude of the nurse to illness? Might it not be very harmful to healthy women to be dealt with by people who had become conditioned to people being ill, who need 'care' rather than just emotional support? Is this, perhaps, why the majority of women in this country who are in labour are actually lying neatly in a bed - the most physiologically undesirable position for them to be in? Why are they lying in bed? This is a position which engenders maternal hypo–tension, fetal hypoxia, less effective uterine contraction and the need for more analgesia as well as failing to utilize the effect of gravity on the descending fetal head.

Is it perhaps because most midwives trained as nurses first?

In this country and in Europe it has always been possible to train as a midwife from the start of training and not to train as a nurse first. The training is longer than post-RGN qualification - it is a period of three years in this country at the moment. But unfortunately there is only one midwifery school doing the direct entry training now, and there are about six applicants for every place.

We need to rethink our training of midwives. I'm glad to say that we are - both the Royal College of Midwives, the Association of Radical Midwives and the midwifery committees of the UKCC and the national boards. Are you thinking about it too? Isn't it time other midwifery training schools took the initiative and began training people who want to be midwives without training them to be nurses first? Or perhaps I'm wrong. What about being chiropodists first? It would be a useful sideline wouldn't it?

Reproduced with kind permission from Nursing Times, February 12 ,1986.

Three Steps Forward

The midwifery profession can congratulate itself on a progressive year, says
Caroline Flint. Here she gives three good reasons why

Let 1985 go down in the annals of midwifery history as a Very Great Year for midwives. Three momentous things happened for the profession during these months.

First, the English National Board's strategy document on professional education/training courses is probably the best news midwifery education has heard in years. Many midwives have been saying for some time that it is inappropriate (and very wasteful) for midwives to train as nurses first and midwives subsequently. The basis of nurse training at the moment is that the student is taught to look after the sick and make them healthy. But midwives rarely have sick people to look after - we assist healthy women and their families through a normal physiological process - and by putting them in a sick role, can actually do them harm.

For example, a woman who labours in bed may be restricting the pelvic diameters, causing maternal hypotension which in turn, because of pressure on the ascending aorta and the inferior vena cava leads to fetal distress. Labour may also be slowed down, as the tendency of gravity to accelerate the descent of the fetal head and to stimulate cervical dilation does not happen when the woman is lying flat. ·

When one has trained as a nurse and works in a hospital with labouring women it is difficult not to treat these women as 'ill' - to mother them, to put them to bed and call the doctor to decide how they should be treated. When we are dealing with labouring mothers, people who are taking on the greatest responsibility of their lives, it is important that they should be treated as adults. We should listen to them and let them make decisions about the birth of their baby. Midwives need to be assertive and stand up for women (and their partners). Sometimes they may even need to protect them from the consequences of being in hospital.

The new ENB strategy document pleases vocal groups who have been clamouring for more direct entry training for midwives. The document describes an imaginative range of common core subjects to be studied during the first year. Health promotion, health maintenance, social policy and administration, epidemiology, inform–ation technology and liberal studies. These topics will reinforce the vision of healthy, responsible adults and help students to grow into equally healthy responsible adults.

If these proposals are accepted, it may mean less wastage of midwives. At present, for every midwife who practises there are four qualified midwives who do not. A survey is being carried out to establish why midwives leave the profession in droves. Perhaps you know someone who has left midwifery?

The second important development for midwifery in 1985 was the inauguration of MIDIRS, the Midwives Information and Resource Service. This visionary project aims to raise consciousness and the level of knowledge of midwives. MIDIRS will send information packs out to individual midwife members three times a year - a bumper bundle of research findings, new initiatives in midwifery and information that the well-informed midwife needs to know. The service is also planning to have in-depth 'fact packs' on specific subjects such as artificial rupture of membranes, acceleration of labour and the third stage of labour. Other plans include computer literature searches and a research liaison centre.

The third exciting happening in the world of midwifery in this year is the publication of an international journal for midwives, *Midwifery*. The subscription is £21.50 for four issues a year (special rate for RCM members). There is an international news section, information on the International Confederation of Midwives, papers from midwives and features on different specialities from around the world.

Some years I wonder where midwifery is going. Some years I think we have taken three steps backwards, but this year I feel the profession is alive and well - and getting better and better informed. What will 1986 bring?

References

Dunn, P. (1976). 'Obstetric Delivery Today. For better or worse?' *The Lancet* 1; 7963, pp.790–93.

Flynn, A.M., Kelly, J., Hollins, G., Lynch, P.F.(1978). 'Ambulation in Labour.' *British Medical Journal* , 2; 6137, pp.591–93.

Reproduced with kind permission from Nursing Times, September 11, 1985

Symbols of Servility

Skimpy national uniforms and 'pretty' caps can be a positive barrier between the midwife and the family, argues Caroline Flint

Half of Tooting has seen my knickers. This dubious privilege is not earned, sought after, or even desired by most of its recipients. Even when wearing my Christmas pairs (one pair with sprigs of holly, one with snow flakes, one with Father Christmases and one with a Happy Christmas motif), it is a view that few, even my nearest and dearest would cross oceans for. Who are these less than lucky people who have been subjected to this sight? What common denominator unites them? They are the people whose babies I have delivered.

Probably in the heat of the moment, many of these parents have thought that this vision was a momentary lapse, or a refined type of distraction technique for strong labour. But, I am sorry to relate, this vision occurs every time I sit down on a low stool, whenever I squat to deliver a woman in a similar position, and frequently when I bend.

I am a proud member of the greatest and perhaps the most influential of all historical professions - I am a midwife. As a professional woman why am I not dressed in clothes that befit my calling? As a woman who wants to retain credibility, why am I exposing myself to ridicule and embarrassment? The sad reason is that I am employed by the National Health Service which, in its wisdom, has seen fit to rig me out in the uniform of another (and different) profession – the uniform of a nurse. Nurses' uniforms look fine on nurses; to my jaundiced eye most nurses are young and fairly slim. Most midwives are women of mature years and even maturer figures. As a midwife with a decidedly comfortable figure, wearing the skimpy garment which is known as 'the national uniform', I am daily subjected to the embarrassing knowledge that the people of Tooting are getting a very strange impression of my profession.

As long ago as 1978, in a letter to *Nursing Mirror*, it was stated that proper lifting techniques are impossible because of the narrow width of the nurses' uniform skirt.[1] In the report of an RCN working party entitled *Avoiding Low Back Injury Among Nurses*, recommendation 14 suggests that a trouser suit should be incorporated into the uniform to avoid low back injury in nurses lifting patients.[2]

If nurses' uniforms are not even very useful for nurses, how much less useful are they to midwives? Midwives who are forever helping labouring women up the bed, demonstrating different delivery positions, delivering babies in different positions, sitting on low stools in the delivery room. A skimpy skirt is probably the least useful article of clothing we could ever wear. If there is some strange reason for dressing midwives in the clothes of another profession, we would probably fare better if we wore the green boiler suits that the engineers and plumbers wear in the health service.

A consultant paediatrician once answered my grumbling about being dressed in the clothes of another profession by telling me that everyone in his hospital knew who he was without a uniform, and he went on to add that he never wore a white coat. He looks like a professional without either uniform or white coat - of course he does - he wears good clothes and he walks with confidence in the same way that most professional people do. I do not wear good clothes and frequently do not walk with confidence because my purse is about to fall out of the skimpy national uniform, or my tights which are obligatory with the national uniform, have laddered for the hundredth time.

There are times when I look like a professional. These are the times when I wear my own clothes. My clothes are designed for me; they are my taste and I buy them in colours that suit me. In my clothes I look like me. As Ann Rider said at this year's annual meeting of the Royal College of Midwives, the role of the midwife in the postnatal period has changed from that of a physical carer to that of educator, counsellor and supporter of the family in the changing relationships within the new family. The new family is not helped by the barrier that my national uniform creates between us: they need to see me and we need to relate to each other as people.

If some of my midwifery colleagues want something to cover their own clothes, what about taking on the garment that so many doctors are abandoning, the white coat? These are useful overalls that many professions use - dentists, greengrocers, vets, hospital receptionists, medical students, pharmacists and the specimen porter; how about midwives too?

If we decide to take on the green boiler suits or white coats to enable us to practise more effectively and to prevent us displaying our underwear, what will we be doing with our caps? These fluffy bits of lace are neither more nor less than symbols of servility.

Why do I call these caps, beloved of so many of my colleagues, symbols of servility? If you open out many of the caps of the great teaching hospitals you will discover that the frills and ruffles are embellishments to what is, in essence, a Victorian maid's cap, which started life as a cover for her hair and is now merely an ornament serving no practical purpose. When I write these words I can hear the cry go up, 'But they're so *pretty*, and I cannot help but agree. My own particular cap is very 'pretty', but as a professional woman is my aim really to look 'pretty'?

My cap takes an hour to make up. It has to be starched, ironed, stitched with running stitch, moulded around a saucer and the requisite number of ruffles put in it. It is a chore to be put off, done once a year or delegated to a friend. As a professional woman dealing with the public, I need to be careful about cleanliness. Consequently I wear a clean dress every day, clean bra, clean tights and the aforementioned articles to be viewed by the world, clean every day. I also shower and wash my hair every morning. So I set off for my work spanking clean and fresh, except that on my clean head I wear a very dirty cap, because of the time and toil involved in making it up.

My cap becomes dirtier throughout the day. In the delivery ward I brush it against the big light; when delivering a baby to a woman in a semi-squatting position I brush it against the labouring woman; when bending down to get something out of a cupboard I brush it against the top of the door. My symbol of servility is not very hygienic.

My symbol of servility is not very practical, either. It does not cover the hair or show evidence of training or of special midwifery skills. How can it, when it is worn by waitresses in motorway cafeterias, assistants in supermarkets and untrained care personnel? If my symbol of servility was anything other than what I describe it, why don't other professionals rush to take it on to enhance their status? Imagine your professor of obstetrics in my frilly cap. Does she/he want to look 'pretty'? Or your solicitor? Or your accountant? Who will rush to take on my cap when I am allowed to discard it, together with my national uniform and when I am allowed to dress as my profession needs me to? Midwife means 'with woman'; I suggest that means wearing my own clothes.

References

1. Letters. *Nursing Mirror* .1978; 146:12.
2. The Royal College of Nursing (1979).
Avoiding low back injury among nurses. Royal
College of Nursing, April.

*Reproduced with kind permission from Nursing
Times, October 10, 1984*

Childbirth Attitudes

The six articles comprising 'Childbirth Attitudes' were written between 1982 and 1986 and encapsulate what people love and hate about Caroline's writing, namely her effusiveness, her ability to ground her arguments in the realities of her clinical practice, her eclectic use of research, her willingness to embrace controversy and her tendency to sacrifice subtle complexities for what she sees as the fundamental truth.

The title of the earliest piece 'The Obstetrics of Fear' is polemic and the opening sentence is couched in language counter to the traditions of 300 years of empiricism. Neither is likely to convert her antagonists to the arguments in the article. So to whom is the article addressed? Caroline has mainly written for one audience: those who are unhappy with the 'status quo' in maternity care and aware that there are many areas in it that are substandard or could be vastly improved. Caroline has the ability to articulate, and make public, issues which have concerned, irritated, excited, frustrated and saddened midwives and others throughout the United Kingdom. When she says in 'The Obstetrics of Fear' that midwives have 'been intimidated into thinking that (their) feelings are irrelevant and unscientific' she is inviting us to create a new discourse about maternity care with her, appealing through her illustrative use of her own practice to what we have felt or thought but too often have been unable to say. Caroline's very public refusal to be intimidated, together with her ability to persuade editors to let her have column inches, has played an important part in reformulating the agenda for maternity care over the last 10 to 15 years.

The theme of this section is attitudes: attitudes to childbirth, attitudes to women, to women's bodies and implicitly attitudes to life itself. Caroline's own approach to midwifery and her beliefs about the direction it should take are constantly framed against the backdrop of her personal life. Midwifery should facilitate not only the birth of babies but also the birth of mothers with the emotional imperative to mother with confidence and pleasure. Her own experience of being mothered ('The Obstetrics of Fear') and of being a mother acts as a catalyst for her vision for maternity care.

'Mother and Midwife – on the same side' is also interwoven with autobiography. In 1970, long before she qualified as a midwife, Caroline became an antenatal teacher for the National Childbirth Trust and has continued to run NCT classes ever since. The title 'Mother and Midwife' and the partnership between midwives and women argued for in the article reflect the unity of experience and purpose in Caroline's personal and professional life. The myriad of ways in which our personal histories and professional lives interconnect has yet to be studied seriously but Caroline has never subscribed to the ideal of the 'detached professional': the detached midwife being a contradiction in terms is indeed her theme.

Some people do not like Caroline (nothing personal you understand – they just don't like what she stands for or how she stands for it). It is hard for midwives to be assertive and seeing, hearing or reading of others assertiveness can be an uncomfortable experience. It is perhaps Caroline's misfortune that influencing people and winning friends are not always as closely connected in reality as in popular literature. The hapless houseman in 'Nowhere Else to Go' understandably may have come to regret opening his mouth in front of her but I doubt his attitudes escaped unscathed. The professional members of the Maternity Services Liaison Committee in 'We Always Do That Here' may have deleted her from their Christmas card list but probably introduced a smidgen of self-criticism to their subsequent agendae. There are sufficient midwives for whom being liked (by the consultant, the registrar etc.) ultimately takes precedence over standing up for clients to make Caroline and others like her even more necessary and refreshing.

Caroline's assertiveness is not just a paper exercise. In the early 1980s a new wing was built at St George's Hospital and a vast new canteen was opened for *all* staff. After some months of these egalitarian dining arrangements, it was announced that an adjacent room would be opened as a smaller dining facility with waitress service. (Meals would cost ten pence extra therein.) The consultants flocked towards the waitresses with everyone else keeping a respectful distance. It may not have been called a Consultants' Dining Room but everyone understood the intention. They reckoned without the antenatal clinic sister. Caroline was having none of this nonsense and, rounding up any hungry midwife she could find, would persuade them that ten pence was a price worth paying for a classless society and lead them cheerfully into this bastion of medical privilege. There she would plonk herself at tables already occupied by various consultants (just to make sure that there wouldn't be 'consultant tables') and engage them in prandial chit-chat. Being an occasional visitor to St George's (I worked in its sister unit) I was rounded up for lunch on two or three occasions. Even this little stab of assertion took some nerve. Attitudes and the behaviour they engender are very deeply engrained; which is why most of these articles, written a decade or more ago, could have been written yesterday. Most...but not all: attitudes are slowly changed.

Blue for a Boy

By Caroline Flint. Midwifery sister at St George's, Tooting

I've just visited Thomas' bedroom; it has a blue door, Thomas the Tank Engine pictures all over the walls, blue wallpaper and blue curtains. On the cot is another Thomas the Tank Engine picture and pinned above the cot are a pair of tiny football boots - it's a beautiful nursery for a baby boy. A baby boy who has been dreamt about, welcomed and anticipated.

Thomas' father comes from a family which has few males in it. He was the youngest of five, all the others were girls. Thomas's mother is an only child, so they were both absolutely thrilled when they were told that they were having a boy when she was being scanned when she was 18 weeks pregnant.

At first they decided to tell no one the sex of the baby they were expecting, they kept it as a luscious secret. They planned his name and thought and dreamt about what they would do as their little boy grew bigger. Quite soon though, they couldn't resist telling their parents and their friends, because they knew the baby's sex they were no longer expecting a 'baby', they were expecting Thomas, their son.

I went to see Thomas' bedroom - and in it was Samantha. Thomas had never existed. It hadn't been a baby boy; when she was scanned it was actually a baby girl and the scanner had thought he had seen something which obviously couldn't have been there.

How are Thomas' parents? Because that's who they still are three weeks after delivery. They are pleased and happy that Samantha is well and healthy. They are trying hard to love her and care for her well - the fact that she is a very wingey baby doesn't help, and the fact that she doesn't feed easily also poses problems.

Identity

These parents were expecting a baby boy who had a name and an identity. Despite the fact he never really existed - to them he became a very real small person - they fell in love with a baby son.

Thomas' parents have made me think so much about what we do to pregnant parents in 1986. How, even with the best intentions we mess up pregnancy and childbirth. Thomas' parents went for a scan at 18 weeks of pregnancy, at that time they were expecting a baby - a welcome, looked forward-to-baby. They didn't really mind whether it was a boy or a girl but Thomas' father always secretly hoped for a son and he was over the moon when he learnt that it was.

The obstetrician scanning the mother didn't mean to cause problems when he identified the sex of the baby. He's rather a dab hand at scanning and he often tells parents the sex of their expected baby - usually he's right.

Thomas' parents are in quite a state, they are akin to the parents of twins when one of those twins is stillborn. Their emotions are mixed; they are being torn in two and they are grieving for a child who only ever existed in their minds. They are trying to ignore that grief because they know that he never existed, that it had been Samantha all along.

Ultrasound scans are very useful for locating the placenta, for identifying fetal abnormalities and for dating the fetus when the woman isn't sure of her dates. Samantha's mother was always sure of her dates, she didn't really need a scan to date her baby. There was never any query about it - except that at the hospital she was going to all women are scanned to 'date' their babies, despite the fact that half of the women are sure of their dates. Do we think they are lying when they tell us their LMP or do we just not trust them?

Information

As a tool of modern obstetrics it can be extremely useful when it is used with responsibility, but when it is used for all, indiscriminately, and when it is used to divulge information which wasn't sought, how useful is it then? Is this a responsible way of caring for pregnant parents? Have we made their pregnancy and birth safer? Happier? Have we produced a child of 'better quality?' Or are we just playing with people's lives and emotions?

Something else we have encouraged parents to do is to present themselves for antenatal care early in pregnancy. To this end it is normal for women to have a pregnancy test after missing a period. Pregnancy is acknowledged very early and relatives are told, preparations are made, emotional adjustments begin.

Ten years ago women didn't expect to go to their doctor to discuss their pregnancy until they had missed three periods. Until they were well into their pregnancy. Does the wholesale and indiscriminate encouragement of *all* women to present early in pregnancy really help them?

Does it not perhaps make pregnancy even longer for the parents and their families? Does it perhaps increase the grief of miscarriage when the pregnancy is real and tangible rather than just a lovely secret?

Obviously if the woman wants to terminate her pregnancy the earlier she comes, the better. If the family has an inherited abnormality she should be encouraged to present early, but all women, always? Does it really help? Who does it help? Does it produce better stronger mothers and babies? Happier and more loving mothers?

Pregnant women are individuals, with individual needs, perhaps to treat them all exactly the same may not be in their best interests. Perhaps we play God too much - it's much easier if we just look at this woman and plan her care with her.

She is the person our interest should revolve around and she is the person the care should be based on. Do routine procedures/ routine iron supplementation/ routine scans/ routine monitoring/ routine syntometrine/ routine staying in bed for six hours after delivery/ routine anything really help this individual pregnant woman?

Well do they?

Reproduced with kind permission from Primary Health Care, February, 1986

The Obstetrics of Fear

Pregnant women are sensitive to every word, gesture and expression, says Caroline Flint. She explains how midwives can bolster a pregnant woman's confidence in herself and her ability to mother and be a mother

As a woman, a mother and a midwife, I feel and 'know' many things deep in my soul. Although this may not be as impressive as scientific evidence, those involved in childbirth often recognize that birth is mainly a spiritual experience albeit physical.

One of the crucial issues in midwifery today is that midwives have lost their instinctive and intuitive feelings about childbirth. They have been intimidated into thinking that these feelings are irrelevant and unscientific. They are amazed and delighted when these aspects of childbirth are revealed to them, sometimes by lay midwives with no formal training.

Midwives working in the obstetrics of fear are surrounded by the pathology of childbirth, 'high risk women', intrauterine growth retardation, weight loss in pregnancy, uncertain dates, large or small for dates, and low oestriols. Contrary to this, in July 1981 Macvicar[1] said, 'Obstetric practice should become easier since there are fewer mothers in the so-called high risk groups. Four out of five births now occur to mothers between 20 and 35 years. Before the age of 20 years, social factors tend to increase their risks of pregnancy, whereas after the age 35 years, medical complications such as hypertension and diabetes are more common.'

I was reminded recently of our concentration on the pathological as I was taking a woman's booking history. When I asked about her last pregnancy, her eyes opened wide and she said, 'Oh sister, I had a lot of problems, it was a very worrying pregnancy.' When I enquired further, she said 'Well, I had intrauterine growth retardation and I had 14 scans and it was altogether a very anxious time.' Then I asked how much her baby had weighed at birth. She answered, '8lb 12oz'.

Hall, Ching and MacGillivray[2] pointed out in their paper on routine antenatal care: 'Another problem is over diagnosis: for every case of intrauterine growth correctly predicted by the clinician, there were 2.5 false positives, and for every genuine case of pre-eclampsia or hypertension diagnosed another 1.3 were false positives.'

Pregnancy is a period of heightened sensitivity, a time of transition from one state to another. Pregnant women are sensitive to every word, gesture and expression. Kitzinger[3] describes this vividly. 'The expectant mother is particularly sensitive to any suggestion that things may not be quite as they should be. She stores each word in her mind uttered by the obstetrician when he examines her. Since these tend to be few and far between, it is not difficult to remember what he said and to go home and brood over their exact significance'.

Much current practice encourages pathological responses from the women we are trying to help through the transition to motherhood.

What does motherhood mean? What does it mean to be a pregnant woman? What does it mean to a midwife? What does it mean to a child? What does it mean to you?

If we look at our feelings towards our own mother as children, we discover much about the nature of motherhood. Our mother knew everything, we thought. She was as rich as Croesus, she had the power to buy whatever we wanted. If she would not buy it, she was being difficult, unfair or mean. Her power extended throughout life. Not only could she provide our wants, it was she who said that bedtime was now, it was she who would not let us put our fingers in the lovely holes in the electricity sockets. When we were tired or sad, it was she who cuddled us on her lap and loved us better. It was she who taught us the delight of having a clean, dry, powdered body after a bath. It was she who taught us to love and respect ourselves, who showed us by her love that we were worthwhile and special.

Confidence

What does a mother need to give all this to her child? She needs confidence in herself as a person and a woman, and in her ability to mother. She needs to feel valuable as a person and successful as a woman. She needs to feel confident in her ability to cope with her child, to know that the child is hers, her responsibility, that it depends on her.

For antenatal care to be worthwhile, it must help a mother to feel confident in herself and her ability to mother and be a mother. It needs to increase her self-esteem.

When 130 women are herded together into an antenatal clinic, their self confidence and self-esteem feelings are actually decreased. A woman is shown that she is not special, that she is just one of hundreds and that the clinic staff care so little about her comfort that they leave her sitting for two or three hours with countless other women in exactly the same condition.

The National Childbirth Trust report, entitled 'Change in Antenatal Care' starts: 'The expectant mother is treated as the passive object of management, who is fed into the system and whose progress from point to point is controlled as if she had no wishes or preferences of her own...Clinics are often grossly over crowded and have the atmosphere of a badly managed cattle market.'

The Social Services Committee [4] also refers to 'the cattle truck atmosphere of antenatal clinics'. It recommends that 'steps should be taken to make better use of the midwife in maternity care - particularly in the antenatal clinic (and labour ward) where they should be given greater responsibility for antenatal care of women with uncomplicated pregnancies...Antenatal clinics should be given a more congenial and supportive atmosphere by reducing the number of patients attending, by selecting staff - particularly receptionists and the clinic sister - who are welcoming and by improving the physical facilities and decoration of the clinics.'

The physical position of women throughout antenatal and intrapartum care in most obstetric units is horizontal. It is difficult for even the most articulate woman to think rationally, discuss, negotiate and inquire in such a disadvantageous position. A woman, horizontal or vertical, needs positive reinforcement of her ability to be a mother.

Women are often examined in silence and at speed. Interest is only shown when they present some pathological symptom such as 'I haven't felt my baby move since Tuesday'.

To increase a woman's self-confidence, we need to give positive encouragement and know her as a person. This can only be done by providing some degree of continuity of care, through the use of more flexible working days and by giving an expectant mother opportunities to talk, sitting upright and wearing her own clothes. Horizontal women do not feel in control of their situation and it is not helpful to their concepts of their own value and self-worth.

How can midwives increase a woman's confidence in herself and her ability to mother and be a mother in the labour ward?

In the obstetrics of fear, concern is expressed for the baby's safety during labour. This is a valid and commendable concern but, when overemphasised, can indicate to a woman that her body is a place of danger to the baby. The phrase 'We'd better get this baby out' is used by obstetricians and midwives who see themselves as saviours of the baby - at risk from its mother's body. This is not conductive to helping a woman feel confident in her ability to be a mother. Although a baby must sometimes be delivered at speed, if obstetricians and midwives can be with the mothers as carers, rather than saviours, of the baby the emphasis is much more positive for the mother.

A woman needs to be able to trust medical attendants during labour so she can concentrate without attempting to form new relationships, and so she can relax, sure that everyone present knows what she wants of her labour.

This can be achieved by discussing labour during pregnancy, taking note of a woman's wishes and hopes for labour, and by giving her constant encouragement throughout labour.

Dorsal position

The horizontal position of women in pregnancy is more important during labour. Dunn[5] in an article published in *The Lancet* in 1976, described the advantages of the dorsal position for both mother and baby. These included fetal distress caused by compression of the inferior vena cava and aorta, narrowing of the birth canal and constriction of the pelvic diameters because of the pressure on the sacrum and loss of mobility, less efficient uterine contractions, slower labour and increased pain. Fearing the pain of labour, we may be too eager to urge a woman to have an epidural or pethedine although, for many women, the most effective form of pain relief can be the support and encouragement of a known and trusted midwife. Modern methods of pain relief are useful and effective but one has only to see the pride, delight and feelings of triumph exhibited by a woman who has overcome this gruelling physical experience with her own resources to see that while pain relief must

be available for those who would like it, it may not be constructive to offer artificial forms of analgesia as a first resort.

Encouraging words and an offer of distractions during contractions are far more helpful to many women.

In the first fragile postnatal days, how can we help build the new mother? Again, the words used are vital and will be remembered years after midwives will have forgotten the name of the postnatal ward.

Whether a woman wants to breastfeed or bottle-feed she must be helped and encouraged. Mothers who want to breastfeed but end up bottle-feeding often feel inadequate. Maternity unit staff need to look at why it is happening. Staff often think that, in their ward, there is demand feeding but in fact babies are fed to a scheduled time or are only allowed to suckle for a specific length of time.

If a woman's confidence in her ability to cope is to grow, it may be constructive to signify that breastfeeding is a relationship between two people and, like all physical loving relationships, needs to be worked on by the two people concerned, and that a third person may be an intruder. Unlike many midwives, I do not see the midwife's role in breastfeeding as physical supervision but an emotional support. Breast feeding is best learned in an unhurried atmosphere and in privacy.

At the birth of a family, midwives' attitudes are essential to the well-being of the new mother and baby, and to the new father's feelings of involvement and pride. We need to look at and cope with important issues in order to function more effectively as the Central Midwives Board definition of a midwife – 'A person who is specially instructed and qualified to take professional responsibility and to provide care for women during labour, the postnatal period and for the newly born infant up to the 28th day'.

References

1. MacVicar, J. (1981). 'Changing birth patterns during a period of declining births'. *Maternal and Child Health,* July.

2. Hall, M.H., Cling, P.K., MacGillivray, I. (1980). 'Is routine antenatal care worthwhile?' *The Lancet* 2, p.78.

3. Kitzinger, S. (1962). *The Experiences of Childbirth,* Victor Gollancz Ltd.

4. House of Commons, Second report from the Social Services Committee, Session 1979-80. 'Perinatal and neonatal mortality', HMSO.

5. Dunn, P.M (1976). 'Obstetric delivery today: for better or worse?'. *The Lancet,* 1, 790.

Reproduced with kind permission from Nursing Mirror, July 7 1982

Mother and Midwife – on the Same Side

The old debate about 'meddlesome midwifery' goes on, but the protagonists are different today, says Caroline Flint

Since time immemorial midwives have railed against 'men midwives' or accoucheurs. In 1760, midwife Elizabeth Nihell said, they were 'all for speed' and used instruments because they did not have the patience to allow nature to take its course. And Peter Dunn in the *Lancet* in 1976 listed some of the risks of active management of labour as - 'unexpected prematurity; amnionitis and congenital infection, prolapsed cord, antepartum haemorrhage; complications of fetal monitoring; increased maternal stress and pain; complications of maternal analgesia; abnormal or excessive uterine activity/ tone; uterine rupture; precipitate delivery; fetal distress; obstetric delivery; failed induction; Caesarean delivery; birth asphyxia and respiratory distress;hypoglycaemia hyperbilirubinaemia; mother-child separation; long-term handicaps'.

Peter Dunn quoted Professor G.L. Kloosterman who is convinced that 80-90 per cent of women are perfectly capable of delivering themselves normally without any help. 'Spontaneous labour in a healthy women is an event marked by a number of processes which are so complex and so perfectly attuned to each other that any interference will only detract from their optimal character. ... The doctor who is always on the look-out for pathology, and eager to interfere, will much too often change true physiological aspects of human reproduction into pathology.'

Midwife Juliet Willmott wrote in 1980, 'Pregnant women tend to be treated now as if they are ill and doctors have assumed control over normal, physiological labour as well as over the pathological.'

Throughout history two opposing views have been held: nature can always be given a helping hand or nature should only be meddled with in dire emergencies. At one end of the spectrum have traditionally been midwives who are predominantly female and at the other end have been obstetricians who are predominantly male. Often the edges are blurred and people from both sexes are in both camps, but the protagonists have nearly always been the practitioners, the professionals, the midwives and the obstetricians. Now a new voice is joining this debate and the professionals are at one end and parents are at the other.

Parents have been voicing their opposition to 'meddlesome midwifery' for many years. The National Childbirth Trust is nearly 30 years old and the Association for Improvements in the Maternity Services is in its second decade. Both organizations have always championed parents' rights, but during the past two years the voice of parents seems to have become louder and the professions seem to be hearing more clearly what they are saying.

Perhaps it began on April 4, 1982 when 5,000 women gathered outside the Royal Free Hospital to protest against the takeover of technology there and at most hospitals. A petition was sent round and in March 1983, with 12,000 signatures, it was presented to Parliament by the Association for Improvements in the Maternity Services. The petition called for parents' rights in childbirth to be defined in law thus,

That our parental rights be strengthened so that:

1. We choose where and how we give birth to our children;
2. We receive full information about any drugs, tests and interventions during our pregnancies and births;
3. We can withhold our consent to routine-technological interventions if we so decide;
4. We be regarded as primarily responsible for the care and treatment given to our babies.

We believe that these are inalienable human rights which are regularly denied in many British Hospitals.'

The association has set up a 'maternity defence fund' with a view to suing any hospital which carries out any treatment on a pregnant or labouring women without her consent. The rift between the consumer and the professions seems to be wide and deep, but is this the true picture?

I suggest that the maternity services and those employed within them are at the beginning of the most exciting and healthy reforms ever seen inside the health service. It started at the Active Birth Conferences in October 1982 and March 1983 when a total of 5,000 women and men gathered to hear about ways of having babies in a more actively participating way. The exciting factor at both these conferences was the huge proportion of midwives who were there.

The second exciting event was at the annual meetings of the Royal College of Midwives in Colchester in July when the following motion was debated: 'This meeting believes that flexibility and parental choice in care is inconsistent with the professional competence, judgement and accountability of the midwife.'

The conflict was brilliantly illustrated with a series of role plays by two midwifery tutors, Kate Newsom and Sarah Roch, who enacted the dilemma experienced by a newly-qualified midwife when a woman asks her to deliver her in a squatting position which the midwife has never seen before. Another scene showed a midwife pleading with a woman in the second stage of labour to allow her to perform an episiotomy; the audience listened to the sound of the baby's heartbeats becoming slower and slower as the woman adamantly refuses.

The role plays obviously touched many midwives there, judging by the queue to give their points of view, or those who argued with each other over different ways of tackling the problems. But the most refreshing quality of nearly all the comments was the sympathy and feeling of oneness that the midwives showed towards the woman's need to be the decision-maker in her childbirth even if this at times brought her into conflict with the professionals' wishes.

This feeling came over again when the motion was defeated unanimously. Midwives were showing in a positive way that they are as their Anglo-Saxon name implies - 'with women'.

Women are calling for a recognition that the birth is theirs and that the responsibility for the baby is theirs too. This has to be accepted when we consider that the woman and her baby are normally under the care of obstetricians and midwives for no longer than 10 days and that the care and nurturing of the child will be the woman's responsibility for the next 18 years. The parents were responsible for the conception; the mother was responsible for what nutrients or toxic substances the baby was exposed to during its life within the womb, and if she used antenatal services, where she decided to have her baby - indeed whether or not she actually went through with that pregnancy.

It must be a nonsense to try and take over the responsibility for that baby during a few hours even if one believes, as do many obstetricians, that these are a very hazardous few hours in a person's life.

Sheila Kitzinger said at the rally outside the Royal Free Hospital, 'Women must reclaim their bodies'. When women reclaim their bodies it does not exclude the midwife. Women look to the midwife for support during normal pregnancy and birth; they see her as the guardian of normal childbirth. As the Central Midwives Board says in *The Role of the Midwife:* 'It appears to be readily acknowledged that the midwife is responsible for the care of normal childbirth, but perhaps one of the main threats to the execution of that role is the practical application of the philosophy that childbirth is only normal in retrospect.'

In midwifery we provide a service that must be geared to the needs and desires of its consumers. When we listen to them we shall be able to provide a safe, humane and individualized service. We can only listen if we provide an opportunity for them to talk to us in a quiet and unhurried setting. The labour ward is not the place to do this; it must be done before or after and the listening midwife must have the means to communicate with her colleagues what this woman and her partner have said. But they are on the same side, mother and midwife, midwife and mother.

References

Association for Improvements in the Maternity Services (1983). *Denial of Parents' Rights in Maternity Care.*

Central Midwives Board for Scotland, Northern Ireland Council for Nurses & Midwives, An Bord Altranais, Central Midwives Board (1983). *The Role of the Midwife* .

Donnison, Jean.(1977). *Midwives and Medical Men.* London: Heinemann.

Dunn, P. M.(1976). 'Obstetric Delivery Today. For Better or for Worse?' *The Lancet,* April 10.

Willmott, Juliet. (1980). 'Specialists in Birth' *Nursing Mirror,* July 17.

Reproduced with kind permission from Nursing Times, October 12 ,1983.

A Midwife's Thoughts on Dignity

Preserving a patient's dignity is dinned into everyone during basic training. But what does dignity mean? Caroline Flint describes what it meant for one woman during labour

I delivered a baby this morning. It was so amusing when the baby, who only had her head out, began to cry; I kept telling her that she could not because she was not able to expand her lungs yet. But baby Joanna ignored what I was saying and went on crying until she was delivered.

Joanna's mother delivered on all fours, completely naked (she had suddenly hurled off her nightdress because she found it constricting), her bottom in the air. In fact for 45 minutes during the labour I never saw the mother's face, only her bottom. Joanna's mother was on all fours on a mat on the floor and she leant her face and arms on a large beanbag and a pile of pillows.

Joanna's mother had intended having an epidural, like she had in her first labour, but she could not persuade herself to get up off the floor and on to the bed because she knew how uncomfortable the bed would be and she would not be able to bear the pain, even for the short time it would take to administer an epidural. She could not get over how comfortable she was on her hands and knees.

After the labour, she sat on the floor with her husband and me, cuddling baby Joanna. She looked at me with shining eyes and said, 'Thank you, Caroline, that was so lovely, so dignified. I really felt in control of the whole thing'. Her words struck a chord in me and I thought about them all day. Here was a woman who had been naked, in a position that can hardly be called dignified, feeling very positively that she had given birth with great dignity and control (which she had). I thought about her first labour which she had told me about. She had had an induction, an epidural, and she had been electronically monitored throughout the labour. She had had excellent pain relief from the epidural and had had a liftout forceps delivery. She had given birth on a bed and had kept her clothes on throughout the labour and delivery. In theory, that labour sounds as if it were much more dignified than this one; dressed instead of naked, no pain so no grunts, no groans or sounds of pushing, a covered woman sitting on a bed instead of a naked bottom with no face, and yet Joanna's mother was ecstatic about the delivery and labour this time. She obviously feels incredibly clever and has grown throughout the whole experience.

Dignity. What is it? Is it keeping women's gowns on them when they feel hot and constricted, is it stopping them making noises that offend our sensibilities, is it sedating them so that they can stay motionless and 'dignified' throughout a hugely physical, abandoned, sweaty, steaming process, or is it giving them their head? Is it handing their labours over to them? Is it sitting back and keeping an eye on the fetal heart occasionally but otherwise trying to keep a low-profile?

We all sat on the floor, on a mat covered by a sheet, while I examined the baby. Parts of the sheet were covered with blood and amniotic fluid. Joanna's mother said to me, 'Isn't this cosy and relaxed?' We must have looked like a group at a rather bloody picnic party, but she was right; it was cosy, it was relaxed, but above all it was dignified.

Reproduced with kind permission from Nursing Times, July 4, 1984.

Nowhere Else to Go

By Caroline Flint, midwifery sister, St George's Hospital, Tooting

The houseman looked down the list on the case notes: no artificial rupturing of the membranes; no epidural; no episiotomy; no routine fetal monitoring.

'If this woman wants natural childbirth she shouldn't have come here' he said scathingly, ' she should go and have her baby behind a bush on Hampstead Heath. Doesn't she realize that in this unit we have a technological approach because of all the high risk women we have here, we can't cater for the nut and sandal brigade as well'.

Something inside my head burst (a blood vessel perhaps?). 'Here is the only hospital which is available to her .This is the district general hospital, there is nowhere else for any woman in this area to go – we have closed all the small intimate units in the area. We have told her repeatedly, and with no basis in fact for the last 16 years, that it is unsafe for her to have her baby at home. We give her no alternative, and when she comes in with a perfectly reasonable set of requests we think she is being deviant – she is in a no-win situation and the situation we have put her in is extremely cruel'.

The houseman was surprised at my vehemence. 'But', he countered,' we are doing it for the safety of the babies, we don't want to take any risks, we only want to monitor her to make sure that there is no fetal distress'.

Monitoring

'I wonder if we really are doing it for that reason' I said. 'The Dublin Trial showed that for women labouring for a reasonable length of time there didn't appear to be any benefits in fetal monitoring, and all other trials have shown an increase in caesarean section rates when routine electronic fetal monitoring is used. Perhaps we are only using the monitors because they are there, because they cost a lot of money and we have to justify the expense'.

'Rupturing membranes too, why should she have her membranes ruptured if she doesn't want them ruptured?'

'Well,' said the houseman, 'it's our policy to rupture them at four centimetres, so that we can see the colour of the liquor, so that we can fit a scalp electrode and so that we can make sure that she progresses well in labour and keeps to the Friedman's curve'.

I went to quote to the houseman Dunn's list of hazards and disadvantages of rupture of membranes, and Kay Mordecai Robson who found that women had a 74 per cent chance of experiencing indifference towards their baby if her membranes had been artificially ruptured. And as for the Friedman curve – did anyone ever expect any other human being activities to conform to a time limit?'

Amicable

I asked him if anyone ever grabbed his fork and began force feeding him because he had taken too long with his lunch; or if anyone banged on his door when he was on the lavatory and insisted that he be 'helped' because he had taken too long; or if ever when he was making love, someone had taken over because he was being too long. We argued together in the small hours, amicably because we are fond of each other. But never really did we find a common ground because where each of us stands is light years apart.

The woman got what she wanted and her labour and delivery went well and happily, but that conversation got me thinking really hard.

What has happened to our maternity services? We try and humanize them but when a woman asks to be treated as the normal healthy woman she is 'different', even 'irresponsible'. Every hospital I ever visit tells me its clients are 'high risk'. What happened to the normal women who , until about 20 years ago, had their babies at home? What about the normal women who until last year went to the little units which have been closed down so rapidly during the recent past?

Have all the normal women stopped having babies? Professor MacVicar in 1981 said that women who were having babies were less at risk than in the past because of less very elderly mothers, smaller families, therefore less grand multiparae, and less unwanted babies because of better contraception and more use of abortion. The type of women who are using the maternity services now means that we should have more 'normal' women. They should be given more choice and less intervention.

Fetal scalps clips, artificial rupturing of membranes, monitoring, episiotomy, epidurals, they all have their place and usefulness – but not for everyone and not for every labour. Each of them must be used with discretion, with respect for that particular woman and her needs.

When people tried to put fluoride in the drinking water there was an uproar – not because it wasn't acknowledged that it might be good for many people to ingest fluoride but because the choice was being taken away. Imagine someone handing out lollies to every passer-by. You might like lollies and take one eagerly, I might like lollies and take one but, as sure as humans are humans , there will be some people who don't like lollies and who won't take one. Thank goodness we have the choice.

Isn't it time we stopped trying to foist all our lollies on all women and gave them a choice? And isn't it time we looked at where all the 'normal' women have gone. Maybe they are the women we have sitting in the hospitals, renamed high risk because we want to use all our gadgets? Or am I just an old cynic?

Reproduced with kind permission from Primary Health Care, July ,1986

We Always Do That Here

By Caroline Flint, midwifery sister, St George's Hospital, Tooting

I can't imagine why women are still complaining about their treatment during childbirth; it must be absolute paradise to have a baby in Britain at the moment. Can there really be any room for improvement at all, here and now, in 1986, surely we've got it right?

You may be asking yourself, has Caroline flipped her lid? Why has this critical old bird suddenly had a great conversion, where are her usual moans and groans? The answer, gentle reader, is that I have been a fly on the wall at a Maternity Services Liaison Committee.

You may remember that the Maternity Services Advisory Committee recommended that these committees should be set up locally, when they produced *Maternity Care in Action*. These were guides to good practice in maternity care and were issued between 1982 and 1985. Each guide - one for antenatal care, one for intrapartum care, and one for postnatal and neonatal care - had a check list following each chapter, which was put forward as a 'plan for action' for each Liaison Committee to follow. As the report pointed out 'progress will depend on co-operation amongst everyone concerned'.

Observer

I went to the Maternity Services Liaison Committee - an observer, no more, a mute figure on the periphery - and I watched and listened. The chairman was an obstetrician, sitting next to him were the two obstetricians from the unit and next to them was the director of midwifery services. A paedia-trician came in late and sat at the same end of the large table.

Before the meeting started the group of 'professionals' buzzed amongst themselves, 'have you heard, John's got his fellowship'. 'I saw old...yesterday, I told him what I think about opening up the consultants' car park to the multitude'. The director of midwifery services tried to come in when she could: when a name she knew was mentioned she would say 'He was a registrar when I first came here' or 'he was a houseman when I was a staff midwife in...'.

At the other end of the table was an assortment of 'lay' people; an elderly gentleman who was there representing a community group, a young mother who had her baby with her, which suckled from time to time and made it almost impossible for her to participate fully in the meeting and a representative from the community health council, a very firm and assertive young woman who had obviously read and knew the documents well.

Checklist

The meeting started and the chairman began to read through the checklist. 'Are elective Caesarean sections always timed to take place when all necessary facilities are available and staffing levels are optimal?' This was discussed with the 'professionals' and it was decided that 'we always do that here'.

I listened with interest, I happened to know that staffing levels in this unit were never 'optimal' they could at best be described as 'least minimal'. The community health council representative referred back to an earlier sentence, 'It is now generally agreed that interventions should be avoided unless there are clear medical implications to the contrary'.

The 'professionals' were annoyed that their clinical judgement was being questioned. They felt that this was not the time and the place, but of course they avoided intervention unless there were clear medical reasons to the contrary. The young mother suggested that medical reasons for intervention appeared to be growing, she was reassured that this was only to safeguard the lives of babies like hers.

The meeting ground on. Every point on the checklist was being done in this unit and not only was it being done, it was being done well. I had at last found the place which was perfect in every way!

The 'we always do that here' syndrome is alive and well in most of our maternity units, it is sister to the 'we don't have the room/the money/amenable consultants/supportive management/the staff' syndrome.

It's interesting how 'high risk' women are becoming. I'm beginning to wonder where all the low risk women have disappeared to, especially at a time when women are on the whole well nourished and are not having huge families, so we have few grand multiparae. Those women who *are* most at risk - the women producing babies which they do not want - are much depleted in number because of better contraceptive facilities and abortion services. Women at this moment should be less at risk than any other generation in the past.

Frequently when I give a talk on the 'Know your midwife scheme' (which aims to provide continuity of care for mothers with four midwives taking on responsibility to care for 250 women a year) someone in the audience tells me, 'We already do that here, we've always done it'. I usually suggest that they could be accused of being selfish, if what they are doing is as they describe why don't they write it down? Why don't they share it with their colleagues?

New ideas

The way we all learn, the way ideas are shared is by writing and talking about them. It is no good having good ideas and keeping them to yourself, the women of Britain need to be benefiting from them. We always need new ideas and suggestions, don't we?

Or perhaps you don't because you are lucky enough to work at a unit where everything is perfect, where the staff are able to say 'We always do that here'. Do the women in your area think it's perfect too?

Reproduced with kind permission from Primary Health Care, September 1986

Clinical Issues

The sorts of clinical issues dealt with in this section are those of the everyday interactions between women and their midwives. The nature of 'ordinary' midwifery practice and the issues it raises have been the focus of Caroline's attention. Whilst American midwives like Ina May Gaskin and Elizabeth Davis have written books and articles exploring the experience of midwifery, British midwives have been slow to examine midwifery through the actual experiences of its practitioners.

Caroline is an exception and her book *Sensitive Midwifery*, published in 1986, had both midwives and mothers as its subject. Midwives are players in the drama of birth and not just the stage managers they seem in other textbooks of the time such as that of Margaret Myles. They may only be the support cast but their personalities, words and actions can have a profound effect on the main characters and are therefore worthy of attention.

In the articles making up this section, Caroline does not divorce clinical practice from its practitioners but always presents the words, actions and attitudes of midwives as integral to her consideration of clinical issues. This is an area in which midwifery has developed further than medicine: in medical journals clinical issues are still treated as though they exist in a realm uninhibited by actual people. Most of Caroline's articles by contrast are peopled – peopled by the women she's cared for, met or heard about, and peopled by her colleagues and herself.

The 'clinical issues' discussed in these articles deal with breastfeeding, breech babies, the spontaneous and artificial rupture of membranes, Caesarean section and postpartum haemorrhage. One article explores the labour ward environment and six explore (under various guises ranging from ethical issues to the risks of HIV infection for midwives) unit policies and guidelines for practice. The criticism of routine interventions in normal labour runs as a thread throughout, particularly electronic fetal heart monitoring, artificial rupture of the membranes, the use of fetal scalp electrodes, restricted mobility and unnecessary episiotomies or vaginal examinations. Privacy for clients and the need for clinical autonomy for midwives, together with greater continuity of care are Caroline's prerequisites for improving both the physical and the emotional outcomes of maternity care.

Caroline is what is often termed 'a physical person'. This can be alarming. Hugging and kissing are an occasional rather than day-to-day part of midwifery care for most midwives and their clients ('Care Plan or Talisman?'), and even Caroline has a touch more restraint in person than in print. Nevertheless the breaking down of lay/professional barriers that hugging and kissing represent are central to her vision for midwifery and not simply a frivolous suggestion to annoy the Disgusted of Tunbridge Wellses of the profession (although they have not been without effect in that quarter).

Two of the articles provoked an outcry when they were originally published ('Ethical Issues Facing Midwives' and 'Postpartum Haemorrhage at Home'). The strong feelings underlying 'Ethical Issues Facing Midwives' are apparent in the language used. The scenarios presented were felt by some to be too extreme and to portray rare examples of the very worst obstetric practice. Caroline was upset by the haranguing she underwent as she felt that there was nothing in the article that had not or did not happen. The incidents cited were based on those directly experienced by her or her colleagues and, whilst the presentation of them in such concentration may have made the article somewhat unpalatable, Caroline had thought that this was some dirty laundry which would benefit from public airing.

The criticism levelled at 'Ethical Issues Facing Midwives' was minor compared with the problems which had arisen earlier that same year following the publication of 'Postpartum Haemorrhage at Home'. Whilst the Supervisor of Midwives directly concerned with the birth in question had a frank but friendly discussion with Caroline about her management of the problem, other Supervisors decided to pursue the matter further. Unable to suspend Caroline from practice for failing to call for medical aid because they had no authority in the area where Jane and Harry lived, a group of Supervisors nevertheless made a formal complaint to the then Investigating Committee of the English National Board for Nursing, Midwifery and Health Visiting (ENB) about the article. They claimed that the article had brought the midwifery profession into disrepute by publicly displaying a disregard for the Midwives' Rules. Caroline was informed only that a complaint alleging professional misconduct had been formally lodged about her in relation to the article and duly spent three months trying to ascertain what the charge against her was. Twenty years of marriage to a lawyer rendered her acutely aware that the whole situation was a travesty as far as the concepts of British legal rights and justice were concerned. As her letters and those of her solicitor made clear, she had a right to know with what she was charged. Caroline was at that time an appointed member of the ENB and having to work closely with some of the bureaucrats implicated in the tardiness and secrecy surrounding the complaint against her.

After three months of tension and anxiety she was informed that it had been decided that there was no case for her to answer. The incident was another shameful episode in the Supervision of Midwifery in the UK. More of the issues surrounding and arising from the episodes are explored in many of the articles in section four 'Rules, Laws, Autonomy and Justice'. The fact that 'Postpartum Haemorrhage at Home' had been a serious and honest attempt to discuss Rule 40 of the 'Midwives Rules' within the context of a not unusual clinical event was largely forgotten, but like many of the other clinical issues covered in this section, is still worthy of current debate.

Responsibility for Practice

What should a hospital midwife be able to do to practise truly as a midwife?
Caroline Flint reports on a discussion with her colleagues

'I want to *practise* as a midwife'.

How often have you heard midwives saying this, how often have you said it yourself?

If we are to practise as true practitioners, as real midwives, what do we hospital midwives need to be able to do? What do you do in your hospital that enables you to practise as a midwife, that others don't do in their hospitals? Some colleagues and I sat down the other day and discussed the things that enable us to practise as midwives. Here are some of our conclusions.

When a woman comes into hospital in strong labour it is essential that a midwife can give the woman some sort of analgesia without having to refer to a doctor to write it up on a prescription sheet; a woman in pain needs analgesia *now*, not in 20 minutes.

In 1983, under section four of the notices concerning a midwife's code of practice, the Central Midwives' Board listed the following which may be carried by midwives: antiseptics, aperients, sedatives and analgesics, local anaesthetic, an oxytocic preparation, agents for neonatal and maternal resuscitation.

Most (but not all) hospitals have 'standing orders' so that midwives can administer up to 150mg pethidine, paracetamol, ergometrine, lignocaine, naloxone and other selected drugs without having them written up by a doctor. Standing orders are useful, but many midwives working in hospital would prefer to be able to prescribe these drugs themselves, as their sisters in the community can. To practise fully as a midwife, midwives in hospital need to be able to administer these drugs without prior reference to a doctor.

It is well within a midwife's sphere of practice to be able to diagnose labour. Are there really hospitals in this country where a doctor has to be called to discharge a woman who has come into hospital in false labour? How do midwives feel about that? What happens? Does the midwife ring the doctor and say, 'Mrs Jones came in 45 minutes ago, but she isn't in labour so I'm sending her home to take two Panadol and try to get some sleep; could you come and confirm this?' How does the doctor confirm this? Does he perform yet another vaginal examination? Does he take the word of the expert in normal labour and write in the notes 'Midwife says that patient is not in labour and is going home'? If so, why does a doctor need to be called at all?

Surely in most hospitals, midwives are deemed to be proficient in diagnosing the onset of labour. Can a midwife properly practise as a midwife if a doctor's confirmation is required in her hospital?

In most hospitals in this country, a doctor (usually very junior) examines a woman before transfer to the community. Frequently the woman has already been examined by a midwife. During our discussion we began to feel that there was no reason why midwives in post-natal wards couldn't transfer women to the care of the community midwives without referring them first to a doctor. Obviously if the woman has an abnormality, or a medical condition such as a deep vein thrombosis, a large and painful haemorrhoid, a third degree tear, then of course she would need to be seen by a doctor first. But otherwise is there any need?

Can a midwife practise as a midwife if her examinations on postnatal women are repeated by a junior doctor within a short time? We have heard that there are hospitals where this is happening and we feel that this must undermine the confidence of patients who have been subjected to the same intimate examination only a short time ago. If a midwife is to be a practitioner she needs to be able to carry out examinations of women with the knowledge that she has the responsibility for postnatal checks and that it is up to her to notice any abnormalities. If several people do the same checks, women get conflicting advice and, because the responsibility has become diffused, no one takes ultimate responsibility and so the patient does not receive optimum care.

The same practice should apply to checks on newborn babies. As a practitioner, the midwife should check a baby at birth and daily, and if she is worried about anything she should refer the baby to a paediatrician. But normally, does a baby need to be seen by a paediatrician more than once following delivery?

At six weeks following delivery, is there any possibility of midwives carrying out the postnatal examination? It would be so useful to know how uncomfortable or not the patient was after one's suturing and to get some feedback on the care that had been given.

To be able to practise as a midwife, the midwife must be able to take decisions affecting normal labour, such as when to monitor the baby's hear electronically, when to rupture membranes artificially and when to perform vaginal examinations. Only she knows how this individual woman is faring during this unique labour and it is important to her patient that the midwife is able to conduct the labour and delivery according to the needs of each individual woman.

If there is a rigid hospital policy that vaginal examinations *must* be done very four hours, or that membranes *must* be ruptured at a certain stage, or that women *must not* eat during labour, this removes the autonomy of the midwife, and prevents her from practising her professional role.

At the same time, it is important that the woman and the midwife are assured privacy. The labour ward should be treated as this particular woman's bedroom while she is occupying it and no one should even enter the room without knocking and waiting outside until being let in. We would never just walk into someone's bedroom in their own home; this should not happen in labour wards, either.

From our discussions, we felt overall, that to be able to practise truly as midwives in hospital, there were several areas where we need to be able to take responsibility for our own practice, and we are hoping that readers will write (*c/o Nursing Times*) and tell us their views. What do we as hospital midwives need to be able to do if we are to practise as midwives? What do you do in your hospital that is helpful to our practice as midwives?

Reproduced with kind permission from Nursing Times, August 1, 1984

Care Plan or Talisman?

A new document designed as a care plan for midwives seems to lack the personal touch so essential to midwifery practice, argues Caroline Flint. Nevertheless, she adds, it is a worthwhile paper for any unit trying to implement the midwifery practice

I have been looking at the All Wales nurse manpower planning committee's publication *Standards of Care*, which is a care plan for midwives written by the midwifery sub group. It is a care plan designed for midwives in any situation.

The document states: 'These guidelines to obtain optimum care and satisfaction for a pregnant woman can best be followed by midwives working with obstetricians, general practitioners and other colleagues'. This irritated me immediately because it seemed to me that this phrase was being repeated rather like a talisman, patting other health professionals on the hand and saying: 'Don't worry, midwives won't ever do anything without you'.

This is the same sort of talisman which repeats 'I believe in the team approach' or 'I believe in continuity of care rather than continuity of carer' or 'Midwives are their own worst enemies'. They are just words, repeated with little thought and absolutely no understanding of what they signify for women, but words, that ensure that no action needs to be taken and everyone can just nod their heads in agreement.

I tried to analyse why this first phrase had annoyed me so much when it is relatively inoffensive, and then I realized. It excluded the woman. The word midwife means 'with women' not 'with obstetricians', not 'with general practitioners', not even 'with other colleagues' and it has to be obvious that the basic principle behind midwifery care is 'that the relationship between mother and midwife is fundamental to good midwifery care' and 'that the mother is the central person in the process of care'.[1] Here on the very first page she had been left out.

I looked further and found that on antenatal care it said: 'The midwife will be responsible for agreeing parameters of good health and well-being and for planning the care to meet and maintain these.' This really was a bad start, but on reading further I began to realize that this had perhaps been a slip. The 'patient' is never referred to again. Every page starts with: 'The woman will be helped to acquire knowledge and skills preparing her for the experiences of labour and motherhood.' 'The woman throughout the postnatal period has her individual care needs identified and develops self confidence in her ability to care for herself and her baby/ babies.' The care from then on revolves around the woman and her needs.

The paper is couched in the jargon which surrounds nursing care plans, but it is the clearest I have ever read and any unit trying to implement the midwifery process need look no further - they could easily just take the whole of this paper and use it.

But sadly this paper takes us no further. It rationalizes and plans care as given at present and for that purpose will be useful to many, but I was saddened that it didn't look towards a more intimate relationship between mother and midwife. Nowhere was the woman encouraged to get to know those who would be caring for her and nowhere was there any thought that it might be possible for women to form a relationship with those she is with during her pregnancy, labour or puerperium.

At each point the midwife, the document said, 'will remember to familiarise the woman with the environment, staff roles, and visiting policies', 'the midwife will encourage a calm, supportive environment' and 'will assess, record and feed back information to the mother as appropriate'. So the midwife is definitely being encouraged to talk to the women and communicate with her - but is that all?

Knowing several members of the team who wrote this care plan, and knowing their loving and caring approach to women, I have to presume that such documents possibly preclude the use of the sort of language with which many of us doing day-to-day midwifery care would feel comfortable. Nowhere does it say 'Hug each other as necessary' or 'Encouraging words are the order of the day here' or 'Rub husband's back if he is getting tired' or even 'Kiss all the family'.

Obviously, this approach is assumed by authors of the care plan, and obviously they would approve and use this approach. But I think they have left out something really important. Midwives using the type of approach described may feel that they are doing something 'wrong' or 'deviant', or may even be admonished because 'that isn't part of our policy'.

But maybe I am being harsh - on page twelve one of the midwifery actions during labour is to 'encourage and engender privacy' and to provide 'emotional support from midwives and the labour ward staff'. Yet even that makes me uneasy - midwives and labour ward staff, how many are we expecting in there? Where is the privacy talked about on the same page?

There are two phrases in the document which amused me After the birth of the baby 'the midwife will place the baby in a cot at the bedside' - no deviant behaviour like cuddling the baby please! And at delivery one of the actions of the midwife is to 'inform the mother of the baby's sex'. Perhaps the women in Wales are more backward than the women in England and don't know the difference between the two, but I doubt that. But I have to say that it's usually the woman who tells me what the sex of her baby is - it's difficult for me to get a look in at that stage.

I've been facetious about some of this document but it would be worthwhile for midwives to obtain a copy - they can get one from East Dyfed Health Authority, Starling Park House, Johnstown, Carmarthen SA31 3HL.

Reference
1. Association of Radical Midwives (1986). *The Vision* Ormskirk, ARM.

Reproduced with kind permission from Nursing Times, October 1, 1986

Artificial Rupture of the Membranes

Time to think again?

In 1976 a group of student midwives met together to form a support group, they were the founders of a group which was to have a significant effect on the future of midwifery and maternity care. They needed a name that fitted the initials ARM because these were the initials of the most common intervention in labour - artificial rupture of membranes.

These midwives, who challenged and questioned every 'routine' carried out on individual and idiosyncratic women, called themselves the Association of Radical Midwives - affectionately known as ARM.

Go into the labour ward in the country and on the board will be the initials ARM written alongside many of the women's names there - artificial rupture of the membranes or breaking the waters remains the most common intervention that women in the UK are likely to experience, an intervention so common and perceived as so 'normal' that statistics of its occurrence are frequently not kept. While we are looking at almost everything done to women in labour and pregnancy, perhaps it is time to look at the effects of this intervention and at actually what the implications are of what we are doing when we perform this most common of interventions.

All interventions in labour have a multiple effect – they have an effect on the length and quality of labour, they often have an effect on the woman's mobility, they often have an effect on the amount of pain she perceives that she is experiencing – this can lead to a change in her need for analgesia.

Interventions in labour have an effect on the attendants to the woman in that having crossed the barrier between 'not doing' and 'doing' something, then the inclination could well be to 'do something more'.

Interventions can affect women's level of fear and if a woman becomes very afraid could this have a direct effect in the fetus? Could this have an effect on the physiology of the uterus? Might it have an effect on whether the uterus contracts efficiently or not?

Last year (1989) the National Childbirth Trust published the results of a survey of 3,000 women who answered questionnaires on the effects of artificial rupture of the membranes. They answered questions on what the effects were, when it was done and how it was done.

This survey (not a scientifically controlled study, but anecdotal) showed that artificial rupture of membranes invariably increases the pain of labour. It also showed that when membranes rupture spontaneously they appear either to rupture at the beginning of labour or before labour actually starts, or at the very end of the labour when women appear to be able to cope with the increase in pain. When artificial rupture of membranes is carried out it is usually done at between three and four centimetres dilation.

Women answering the survey found that they could cope with labour and its pain until their membranes were ruptured artificially, and when they were ruptured the increase in severity and sharpness of the pain was so severe that they needed analgesia following the procedure.

The NCT survey found that those women who were having their babies at home were much less likely to have their membranes artificially ruptured than women delivering in a Maternity Unit – and it was irrelevant whether the woman was having a domino delivery or a regular hospital delivery. Those midwives attending women in home births appear to use little analgesia – most women having their baby at home, if they use any analgesia at all, will use entonox as their form of pain relief, for the rest they moan, sit in the bath, gyrate their pelvis and get through somehow. The women who give birth at home in 1990 may be a self selected group of strong minded women, anxious to avoid analgesia, but maybe the reason that most of them manage to get through labour without analgesia is because their membranes stay intact?

The reasons for performing amniotomy are usually stated as being in order to speed up the labour, in order to see the colour of the amniotic fluid, in order to attach a fetal scalp electrode and in order to introduce an intra-uterine pressure catheter.

As far as shortening labour, Stewart, Kennedy and Calder (1982) showed that women whose membranes had indeed been ruptured did labour for a shorter period (4.9 hours compared with 7.0 hours when the amniotomy was carried out at between two and five centimetres dilation), but that the fetal acidosis reached worrying proportions when the membranes had been ruptured, the study was a small one –68 women, and further study needs to be carried out with women being randomized either into 'for artificial rupture of membranes' or 'to leave membranes intact until the baby is born in the caul' groups. Until that happens let us consider the benefits to the woman and the fetus of speeding up labour.

It may be that women would opt for quick labours if they genuinely had the choice but this assumption may not be true at all. Many women appear to find fast labours extremely painful, rather shocking and extremely difficult to cope with – all the effects reported by the women in the NCT survey about the effects of ARM.

It may be beneficial to the fetus to be born more quickly , but we really have no idea whether it is or not. If one thinks of other physiological functions besides labour which we share with other mammals – eating food, defecating, having sexual intercourse – with none of them is our aspiration 'to speed them up', in fact there is no other human activity when our desired aim is to hurry a normal process.

When a woman's pain in labour is increased, she may need an epidural, the effects of epidurals are often benign and beneficial in their excellence of pain relief, but studies have described lengthening of labour, increased need for intravenous infusions of syntocinon and an increase in instrumental delivery. This may be a perfectly acceptable trade-off for the pain relief afforded to the woman , but if the need for it was only occasioned by our use of artificial rupture of the membranes, are we right to subject a woman to an increased risk of having an episiotomy and greater bruising of the perineal area due to an instrumental delivery? Even more, are we justified in taking away the woman's ability to 'cope with' her labour? Women point it out as being important factor to them in labour, they are inordinately proud of themselves when they feel that have 'coped'and disproportionately upset when they have to resort to analgesics when they had not planned to. The long term effects of this may not be relevant, but Oakley showed in her study 'Transition of Motherhood' that women who felt they had 'coped' in labour started mothering with a more positive attitude to their abilities than women who felt the 'victims' of the birth process. Other 'soft' data which needs to be looked at further was the study by Kumar and Robson which described delayed onset of maternal affection for the baby following artificial rupture of the membranes – 'a woman had a 90 per cent chance of feeling some immediate affection for her baby if she did not have her membranes artificially broken'. A woman having her membranes ruptured artificially had a 74 per cent chance of experiencing indifference towards her baby. The result was unexpected and may have been chance, but if we are intervening in the bonding between mother and infant by carrying out a procedure which is hard to justify and may be being done because 'we've always done it', we really must start thinking about what we are doing.

The desire to view the amniotic fluid may or may not be justified, viewing the amniotic fluid at four centimetres may be useful but probably not if the fetal heart shows no indications for anxiety. The fetal head entering the pelvis may well occlude later passage of amniotic fluid and the sight of meconium stained liquor. On the other hand the meconium may have been passed as a response to the increased pressure on the fetal head occasioned by the artificial rupture of membranes.

Dunn, (1978), describes the beneficial effect of intact membranes when the presence of amniotic fluid ensures an even pressure on the fetus during uterine contractions, those isometric uterine contractions prevent impairment of utero-placental circulation due to retraction of the placental site.

He also goes on to express anxiety at the increasing rates of congenital infections in his Unit, and he questioned whether these were a result of increasing amniotomy and increasing instrumental delivery following epidural anaesthesia (Sixth European Congress of Perinatal Medicine, Vienna 1978).

In many ways it appears that by rupturing membranes as a routine procedure we are rushing in where angels fear to tread, the effects of ARM are legion and obviously we do not know them all. Donald in 1966 said 'No labour is so pleasing and satisfactory to mother and child as when intact membranes are maintained right up to full dilatation ... with very few exceptions, intact membranes mean an intact mother and an intact baby'. Might he have been right?

References

National Childbirth Trust. (1989) *Rupture of the Membranes in Labour, a survey.*

Stewart, P., Kennedy, J.H., Calder, A.A. (1982). 'Spontaneous labour: when should the membranes be ruptured?' *British Journal of Obstetrics and Gynaecology,* January, Vol. 89., pp.39–43.

Oakley, A. (1979). *From here to maternity, becoming a mother.* Penguin Books.

Oakley, A. (1980). 'Women confined, towards a sociology of childbirth'. Oxford: Martin Robertson.

Robson, K.M., Kumar, R. (1980). 'Delayed onset of maternal affection after childbirth'. *British Journal of Midwifery,* 136, pp. 247-353.

Dunn, P.M. (1978). 'Problems associated with fetal monitoring during labour'. *Sixth European Congress of Perinatal Medicine ,* Vienna, 1978.

Donald, I. (1966). Practical Obstetric Problems.

Reproduced with kind permission from Obstetrics and Gynaecology Product News, Autumn 1990.

Babies Presenting by the Breech

In pregnancies where the baby presents by the breech it would seem that most obstetricians insist that women either labour with an epidural in situ and are delivered in stirrups by forceps, or that the women should be delivered by caeserean section. That there are good reasons for this is not disputed, the dangers of being born breech first are well documented, but not all authors agree with each other as to the specific nature or even proportion of the dangers.

Kasule (1985) says 'Breech presentation and delivery are associated with a high perinatal mortality and morbidity. Even when congenital malformations and intrauterine deaths are excluded, the perinatal mortality rate after breech delivery is 3 to 4 times higher than that associated with vertex delivery.' Rovinsky (1973) quoting 86,812 deliveries at the Mount Sinai Hospital, New York, between 1953 and 1970 suggests a perinatal mortality rate of 8 times higher for breech presentation at delivery than for vertex presentation. Rosen (1984) says 'Inherent in the several increased risks to the breech infant when compared with the infant in the vertex position is the knowledge that breech presentations have been associated with a high incidence of low birth weight (about 20 per cent of the population) and major congenital anomalies (as high as 18 per cent).' He then goes on to list the dangers of presenting by the breech as 'trauma, prolapsed umbilical cord, fetal distress and head entrapment'.

As women feel hemmed in by the lack of choice and the insistence of their obstetrician that they either have a caesarean section or are delivered in lithotomy with forceps, some are turning to home birth and delivery by independent midwives. The independent midwife will invariably advise against delivery at home, and some are able to negotiate, either with their local supervisor of midwives or with a local obstetrician to deliver the woman in hospital with ready access to obstetric and paediatric help, but if the woman insists on staying at home according to the UKCC Midwife's Code of Practice 'In a situation where the midwife considers that home confinement is inappropriate and the woman refuses to take the advice of the midwife to receive care in a maternity unit, the midwife must continue to give care and inform her supervisor of midwives'

So the independent midwife forced into this situation has to look at the myths and practices which have grown up surrounding breech births and try to map out a course which will ensure the greatest safety for both baby and mother. She needs to be aware of the attendant dangers and has to examine the most appropriate way to deliver the baby.

The principle theme underlying modern breech management is that for the baby to deliver in this position the dangers to that baby are multiplied and the risk of perinatal mortality is increased. The independent midwife needs to survey the literature (both medical and midwifery) to ascertain the attendant dangers.

Myles (1962) lists the dangers to the foetus as fractures of humerus or clavicle, damage to the brachial plexus caused by twisting the baby's neck and causing Erb's paralysis, ruptured liver caused by grasping the abdomen, damage to the adrenals caused by grasping the baby at kidney level, crushing the spinal cord or fracturing the neck by bending the body backwards over the symphysis pubis while delivering the head.

Collea (1978) mentions the incidence of brachial plexus injuries in vaginal delivery breeches, and Garry (1980) has a very long and depressing list of trauma which the baby can sustain 'intra-cranial haemorrhage from rupture of tentorium cerebelli of falx cerebri, due to rapid moulding, dislocation of shoulder, fracture of clavicle, fracture of humerus, dislocation of neck, Erb- Duchenne paralysis, damage of sternomastoid muscles, prolapsed cord, rupture of viscus usually liver or kidney due to pressures or faulty handling, dislocation of hip joint by traction, fracture of femur in flexing extended knee, genital oedaema, disruption of knee joint and apnoea due to premature separation of the placenta'. Collea (1980) describes the problem of two babies with nuchal arms.

On looking through the literature one learns that although obviously there must be increased danger of the baby's head being trapped at delivery when the cervix is not fully dilated, according to most of the literature the greatest danger to the baby seems to be the trauma caused by the person delivering the baby being over anxious and too rough in their delivery techniques.

As a midwife about to deliver a baby presenting by the breech, I must take cognizance of Russell's work (1982) and I must think rationally about the position which will give the baby the most space in order to be delivered. When one considers the wisdom of having women lying down with their legs in lithotomy stirrups, one can see that although the thighs are abducted in this position the sacrum and coccyx are being pressed upwards and consequently the antero-posterior diameters of the cavity and outlet of the pelvis are reduced. Also the great benefits of gravity on the fundus which would help to keep the head flexed are lost.

With the baby presenting by the breech the head is usually fairly well flexed and the largest diameter to come through the pelvis is the Sub-Occipito Frontal which measures ten cms or the Occipito-Frontal diameter which measures 11.5cms. If the anterior posterior diameters of the cavity and outlet are reduced from their normal 12cms even by one centimetre this can leave very little leeway for a safe delivery. On the other hand if the mother is encouraged to take up a squatting position, Russell(1982) describes an increase in both transverse and antero-posterior diameters of the pelvic outlet. His records observed increases of one centimetre in the transverse, so the diameter which is normally regarded as being 11cms could increase to 12cms, and an increase of two centimetres in the antero-posterior diameter increasing the normal measurement from12cms to 14cms. The same author described in 1969 an increase of 28 per cent between the supine and squatting positions. He also points out the importance of the woman's naturally occurring rocking motion which seems almost universal when women are allowed to labour in an upright position. Dunn (1976) points out the increase in efficiency of uterine contractions when the woman is standing.

White in his Emergency Childbirth Manual (published date unrecorded) says when describing how to help a woman to deliver a breech baby, 'In order to add the weight of the baby to the forces helping delivery, the mother should be assisted to a position on her hands and knees,' he also advises 'hands off the breech' because 'more breech babies die of injuries received at the hands of their would-be rescuers than die of smothering'.

It would appear to make more sense anatomically to deliver a woman standing with abducted thighs or on hands and knees with a consequent enlargement of the pelvis. Odent (1984) describes delivering breech babies in the supported squatting position. He goes on to say 'We would never risk a breech delivery with the mother in a dorsal or semi-seated position'.

A position usually referred to as a 'supported squat', with the woman standing, holding onto her partner and facing away from the attendant,means the baby's face becomes visible so that the nose and mouth can be aspirated – in order to release the nose and mouth the woman needs to tip her trunk forwards to bring her trunk into the horizontal plane – but this necessity is avoided if the woman is kneeling on all fours for the delivery. When a midwife has seen a baby been born in this way the rationale behind Burns Marshall manoeuvre is seen immediately as that which has to be done if the woman is upside down (as she is when in lithotomy) and gravity is not used in order to help the baby's nose and mouth to emerge.

By standing in a supported squat the woman feels more in control of the situation, the attendant needs to remain calm and trust in the woman's ability to give birth. I would not encourage women with babies presenting by the breech to give birth at home, but I would encourage obstetricians to examine the way breech babies are being delivered at this moment and to ask themselves whether this way might not be rational – taking cognizance of the effect of maternal posture on pelvic diameters and the effects of gravity.

References

Collea Joseph V. et al. (1978). 'The rand omized management of term frank breech presentation: Vaginal delivery vs. caesarean section'. *American Journal of Obstetrics and Gynaecology.* Vol.131, pp. 186-195.

Collea Joseph V. et al, (1980). 'The rand omized management of term frank breech presentation: A study of 208 cases.' *American Journal of Obstetrics and Gynaecology .* Vol. 137, Number 2, pp. 235-242.

Dunn, Peter M. (1976). 'Obstetric delivery today. For better or for worse.' *The Lancet.* April 10, 1976.

Garrey, Govan, Hodge, Callender (1980). *Obstetrics Illustrated.* Churchill Living stone.

Kasule, J. et al. (1985). 'A randomized controlled trial of external cephalic version'. Vol. 92, pp.14–18.

Myles, M. (1962). *A Textbook for Midwives.*Fourth Edition. Edinburgh and London: E & S Livingstone Ltd.

Odent, Michel. (1984). *Birth Reborn.* Random House.

Rosen Mortimer, G., Chik Lawrence (1984). 'Study undertaken to determine the effect of the choice of birth route on infant outcome in fetal breech presentation'. *American Journal of Obstetrics and Gynaecology* Vol. 148, No. 7, pp.909–914.

Rovinsky Joseph J. et al (1973). 'Manage ment of breech presentation at term.' *American Journal of Obstetrics and Gynaecology*, February 15, Vol.115, pp.497–513.

Russell J.C.B. (1969). 'Moulding of the pelvic outlet'. *Journal of Obstetrics and Gynaecology of the British Commonwealth*, Vol.76, pp.817–820.

Russell, J.C.B. (1982). 'The rationale of primitive delivery positions'. *British Journal of Obstetrics and Gynaecology* , September, Vol.89, pp.712–715.

UKCC (1983). *Notices concerning a Midwives' Code of Practice for midwives practising in England and Wales.* London: UKCC.

White Gregory J., M.D, *Emergency Child birth. A handbook for policemen, ambulance drivers and Civil Defence volunteers.*

Reproduced with kind permission from Obstetrics, Gynaecology Products News, Summer 1989.

Ethical Issues Facing Midwives

What's in a name? A midwife is different from a nurse

'It's not like that for midwives' I hear myself saying, and I see the nurses raise their eyes to heaven and yet again I have got up their noses, because they are fed up with hearing this refrain from me. At every encounter with nurses, midwives have to restate their position and their identity. The midwives who are on the English National Board have to say it over and over again - it's different for us, we are midwives, not nurses. By repeating it thus they tend to incur the wrath of nurses - by having to reiterate it repeatedly they are impeded from taking their profession forward and concentrating on the matter in hand, they are taking time to establish in other professionals' minds the identity of the midwife. In the past the professional body for midwives was the Central Midwives Board, a separate body, everyone on it knew that the midwife was professionally separate and different from nursing, with separate roots and a separate philosophy and educational structure. This did not have to be spelt out as a preface to every discussion. The Board was able to get on with working out those problems that midwives have as a profession, and to go forward as a profession without interminable debate as to who they were.

Should I let that happen to women?

A huge ethical dilemma for midwives is having to stand by and watch things being done to women which their heart screams out against. A doctor chatting pleasantly over the abdomen of a woman on whom he is doing an amniocentesis - as if she were a frozen chicken. A doctor persuading a woman to have an induction, or persuading her to have a hospital confinement when she really wants a home confinement. A doctor with his hand inside a woman's vagina persuading her to have her membranes ruptured which you know the woman doesn't want; or a doctor doing fetal blood sampling on a baby which is almost crowning; the doctor doing a vaginal examination on a woman and telling her scornfully that she is less than the midwife's estimation two hours ago; the doctor who apparently gets a kick out of doing vaginal examinations and does too many too often - and the midwife feels she can't say anything because everyone will think it's her with a dirty mind and it may be that he is inexperienced and is learning.

Sometimes the midwife feels like a concentration camp wardress, allowing things to happen to women that she wouldn't allow to happen to her sister. However, because she doesn't really know the woman, and because she doesn't want to impose her opinions on the woman, and the doctor is kind and his intentions are that he honestly believes that induction/fetal blood sampling/ARM are the best for her and her baby - the dilemma is great. She ends up standing by the woman and holding her hand - but inside she is feeling that she should be doing something to prevent this happening to the woman.

Practising autonomously

Sometimes a midwife has great difficulty in practising autonomously because she either feels hemmed in by policies which have been drawn up with 'an' average woman in mind, and which do not appear to be appropriate for this woman, or she is given advice based on 'unwritten' policies from midwives more experienced than she is. 'You'd better do it, Miss Francis really creates a stink if she finds you haven't continuously monitored.' 'But there is no evidence to show that it is effective in decreasing the perinatal mortality rate, it just increases the caesarean section rate and the instrumental delivery rate - it said so in the Lancet in December 1987.' 'Miss Francis doesn't read the Lancet, you're just trying to be too clever by half - get on and put the monitors on or you'll be in trouble.'

Tiny babies

Babies born months before the allotted time, at 24 weeks or 26 weeks, arrive into this cold world and are immediately whisked away to have tubes put down their throats, intravenous drips into their tiny hands, electrodes on their delicate skins – they are kept alive for a week, two weeks, even sometimes five weeks and then they die.

The midwife who delivers them wonders to herself – wouldn't it be kinder to the baby and to the parents to allow them to cuddle their baby until it dies, but what if it lives? Her friends in the Neonatal Unit introduce her to two-year-olds who were born at 1.5kg and are now apparently normal. Who is she to decide who should have intensive resuscitation or not? But still her heart is troubled.

This is not the only resuscitation which troubles her – she is a Community Midwife and she takes a woman into hospital with meconium stained liquor during labour. The woman delivers normally with a paediatrician present. The midwife aspirates the baby's mouth and throat very thoroughly whilst the baby's head is out (but the baby is not yet born) and once the baby is out, hands him to the paediatrician. The paediatrician's 'resuscitation' of the Apgar 9 baby is so over zealous that the baby sustains a pneumothorax and has to be in SCBU for five days following delivery. The woman looks at the midwife and says brightly 'It's just as well we came into hospital isn't it? What would we have done at home if the baby had been so poorly?'.

Similarly, a woman having a breech who insists on walking around and refuses an epidural despite great pressure. She eventually succumbs and ends up with a caesarean section under epidural for failure to progress from seven centimetres – fetal heart at all times excellent. The baby comes out crying lustily but, by the time the paediatrician has finished 'resuscitating' him, he is shocked, pale, in need of oxygen and has to be intubated. Everyone turns to the mother and says 'Well it's a good thing you had a section isn't it? The baby wasn't happy in there. Now you know why we suggest that women have epidurals when they are carrying a breech baby. You'll do what we say another time won't you?'.

In such instances what can a midwife do? What can she do when the woman asks her 'What was wrong with my baby, Sister? He seemed fine when he came out.' The midwife knows that no-one has been deliberately cruel or unkind– perhaps over zealous and not aware of their own strength, but what can she do or say?

Screening for fetal abnormality

Some of the tests are not wholly accurate, ultra sound scanning being a case in point. The woman is told that terrible things are happening to her baby – it's too small, it's got a hare lip, it has cysts in its brain. However, when the baby comes out, all is revealed to be normal – but what has happened to the woman's confidence in the child? The relationship between them is damaged. Without the scan (and for the scan read alphe feto protein, chorionic villus sampling etc.), she could have lived in peace with her pregnancy and baby, but because of the false alarm she has been hurt. What does the midwife say when she is asked 'What do you think Caroline? Should I go ahead with this pregnancy?'

Being a midwife is to tread through an ethical minefield and we need to be stronger and braver than is sometimes possible. Perhaps the only guideline we can cling to our name – MIDWIFE – with woman – that is where our loyalties lie.

Reproduced with kind permission from Midwives,, Health Visitors and Community Nurse, Vol. 24 August 1988

Safer Practices

Midwives are concerned about reducing the risks of contracting AIDS.
Caroline Flint suggests that less medical intervention could be the answer

Midwives sometimes express their concern at the danger of catching AIDS from undiagnosed women in labour. And midwives all over the country are now trying to wear gloves at even the quickest delivery while masks are reappearing at a rate of knots. But I wonder if we have given real thought to the problem of AIDS and, for that matter, Australia Antigen or Hepatitis B carriers.

For the midwife, the great dangers from these diseases come from needle stick injuries and from the ingestion of blood or amniotic fluid into the mucous membrane of the mouth, eyes or any open wound that she may have.

We need to look systematically at the dangers of needle stick injuries. For midwives these dangers are very real. They often use two instruments which are the source of many such injuries - the amnihook and the fetal scalp electrode - and they are also at risk when suturing a woman's perineum.

The conclusion I come to is that we must really question the need for indiscriminate rupturing of membranes and indiscriminate application of fetal scalp electrodes and use both instruments with great care. Artificial rupturing of membranes has been under question for many years and the adverse literature is legion.

Caldeyro-Barcia[1] has shown in 70 per cent of pregnancies the membranes do not rupture spontaneously before the end of the first stage of labour. So when we artificially rupture membranes, we are intervening in 70 per cent of women's labours and Dunn[2] lists many adverse effects of artificial rupture of membranes as does Inch[3] in her comprehensive study of all the interventions practised in modern childbirth. Inch demonstrates that labours are shortened by 40 minutes because of artificial rupture of membranes, but there is no evidence to show that a shortened labour is of benefit to either mother or baby. According to Robson[4], the mother has a 74 per cent chance of feeling indifferent towards her baby if her membranes have been artificially ruptured.

Electronic fetal monitoring has been questioned by many, especially in the randomized controlled trial carried out on 12, 964 women in Dublin by Macdonald, Grant and colleagues[5], who showed that there was a greater risk of instrumental delivery when electronic fetal monitoring was used. Nor was there any strong evidence to show that electronic fetal monitoring improved fetal well-being.

If these two procedures can also carry risks for midwives (and doctors), we need to question their routine use. It is a routine which is indiscriminately used in many units. These policies, which have questionable value for women, have undoubted dangers for the midwives and medical staff.

As for perineal suturing, some women will inevitably sustain a tear during the second stage of labour and the condition of some babies will inevitably demand the use of episiotomy. But Sleep at al[6] showed that when episiotomies were restricted to fetal indications only, the number of women who did not need suturing was 31 per cent compared to 22 per cent when a liberal use was made of episiotomy. In other words, when episiotomy was restricted, more women had intact perineums.

What about midwives having open wounds on their hands? Well, midwifery is a stressful job; midwives are paid very low salaries; they experience all the disadvantages that poorly paid workers experience and they are under considerable stress. Like many under stress, some midwives chew their nails and pick at their hands. The way to remove this particular stress would be to do something realistic about midwives' salary structure, but in the meantime the employment of a manicurist on every labour ward or somewhere in the maternity unit would greatly help the promotion of strong nails and unblemished hands among midwives.

We also need to think about the most fundamental issue of all. That is, the only time midwives are in danger of getting amniotic fluid or blood in their mouths or eyes is when the woman is lying at eye-level on a high platform: in other words, on a normal delivery bed in the average labour ward. When the woman is walking about, swaying or sitting in a chair, the amniotic fluid cascades down her legs and on to the floor, and so does the blood and any other secretions. Perhaps this is the time to review our whole practice and, perhaps not surprisingly, we shall find that what women prefer is the same as what is best for midwives. It wouldn't be the first time!

References

1. Caldeyro-Barcia, R., Schwarez, R., Belizan, J.M., Martell, M., Nieto, F., Sabatino, H.,Tenzer, S.M., (1975). 'Adverse perinatal effects of early amniotomy during labour'. In Gluck, L., Chicago, M.L. (Eds.). *Modern Perinatal Medicine.*

2. Dunn, P. M. (1978). 'Problems Associated with Fetal Monitoring during Labour'. Proceedings of the Sixth European Congress of Perinatal medicine, Vienna. Stuttgart: Georg Thienne.

3. Inch, S.(1982). *Birthrights.* London: Hutchinson.

4. Robson, K. (1982).'I feel nothing...' *Nursing Mirror*, Vol.154: 25, pp.24-27.

5. MacDonald, D., Grant, A., Sheridan-Pereira, M., Boylan, P., Chalmers, I.(1985). 'The Dublin randomized controlled trial of intrapartum fetal heart rate monitoring'. *American Journal of Obstetrics and Gynaecology* : Vol 152: pp.524-39.

6. Sleep, J., Grant, A., Garcia, J., Elbourne, D., Spencer, J., Chalmers, I. (1984). 'West Berkshire perineal management trial'. *British Medical Journal,* Vol 289: 6445, pp.587-590.

Reproduced with kind permission from Nursing Times, November 4 1987

Troubled Waters

How necessary is it to intervene medically if a woman has a spontaneous rupture of the membranes when her pregnancy has reached full term? Caroline Flint looks at two studies comparing methods of establishing contractions with no interventions at all

'Pop - it's like a bag bursting inside you.' This is how many women describe the sensation of their membranes rupturing at term, and this, of course, is just what it is. But the implications are far more serious than the mere popping of a paper bag. So often, in the modern labour ward, spontaneous rupture of membranes means that the woman will be admitted immediately, monitored continuously (with all the limitations that implies as far as mobility is concerned, and given intravenous syntocinon within a very short time - immediately in some units, within 4 or 12 hours in others, while some have an even more *laissez - faire* attitude.

As long ago as 1975, Sheila Kitzinger suggested that women having intravenous syntocinon had very painful contractions and were more likely to need analgesia than those experiencing normal ones, that they had more instrumental deliveries, and their babies needed more resuscitation and were more frequently admitted to special care baby units.[1] So, for most women, spontaneous rupture of the membranes means the whole panoply of modern medical intervention. And that, for women hoping for the minimum of intervention, is very disappointing.

But are the dangers from spontaneous rupture of the membranes really enough to justify such a high level of intervention? Most of the literature concentrates on the premature rupture of membranes, with a fetus of less than 37 weeks' gestation, and of course these babies have all the added hazards of being pre-term and need special handling. But what about the woman with a good-sized, apparently healthy baby inside her? Most papers don't seem to address the need to do something about spontaneous rupture of the membranes when there are no contractions; rather, they compare the efficacy of prostaglandin pessaries with syntocinon at establishing regular contractions and come to the conclusion that, whereas protraglandin does stimulate uterine contractions, syntocinon is more reliable.

Two studies actually look at whether it is necessary to intervene - the first was carried out in Bristol[2] when women with ruptured membranes at term who were not having uterine contractions were induced at 9 am the morning after admission. This mean that women admitted at 10 am had 23 hours to wait before being induced, and, interestingly, 105 of the 135 women went into spontaneous labour while they were waiting. Seventy-nine percent of the women went into labour within 12 hours of their membranes rupturing and all but 5 per cent had gone into labour within 24 hours.

Those who had gone into labour spontaneously had a 90 per cent chance of delivering normally. In Bristol, the policy was to augment labour if cervical dilation was not keeping to a specific pattern and 60 per cent of the spontaneous labour group ended up having syntocinon. They had a 49 per cent chance of delivering normally and 41 per cent chance of having a forceps delivery. When women were induced with syntocinon they had a 56 per cent chance of having a normal delivery, but 27 per cent chance of having a Caesarean section.

None of the women going into spontaneous labour needed a Caesarean section, and the authors reported that when the women had waited up to 24 hours there was no evidence of infection in either the mother or the baby. The authors concluded that to wait up to 24 hours before inducing healthy term primigravid women was more advantageous to them than inducing them sooner.

The other study[3] was a randomized control of 134 women with rupture of the membranes at term, but no uterine contractions. They were divided into two groups - in one the mothers were induced with syntocinon if labour did not establish within 12 hours of membrane rupture, while the other group were put on bed-rest. They had their temperatures taken every six hours, to observe for infection, but otherwise just sat and waited.

The group on bed-rest had shorter labours than those in the induced group, who not only had longer labours but more Caesarean sections; in addition they had more intra-amniotic infection than the group of women who were left alone. Over half the Caesareans were for failed induction.

The authors of this study came to roughly the same conclusion as the Bristol authors - that intervention in spontaneous rupture of membranes at term in the absence of uterine contractions has very serious implications and is not necessarily in the best interest of women or their infants.

The other point that come over from these papers is the effect of syntocinon. Sheila Kitzinger was right in her survey when she suggested that having syntocinon means women need much more analgesia and that they have a greater chance of having an instrumental delivery.

With the increasing use of labour ward protocols which use syntocinon to accelerate any labour which deviates, even if only mildly, from the norm, perhaps it is time to look at the use of syntocinon and whether it is being overused. Perhaps a more critical look should be taken at whether labour, which is a normal physiological function, is really being improved by the level of intervention at present in use.

References
1. Kitzinger, S. (1975, 1978). *Some Mothers' Experiences of Induced Labour*. Submission to the DHSS from the National Childbirth Trust. London.
2. Conway, D.I., Prendiville,W.J., Morris, A., Speller, D. C. E., Sirrat, G.M. (1984). 'Management of spontaneous rupture of the membranes in the absence of labour in primigravid labour at term'. *American Journal of Obstetrics and Gynaecology* ; Vol 150: pp. 947-51.
3. Duff, P., Huff, R.W., Gibbs, R.S. (1984). 'Management of premature rupture of membranes and unfavourable cervix in term pregnancy.' *Obstetrics and Gynaecology* ; Vol 63: pp. 697-702.

Reproduced with kind permission from Nursing Times, November 26, 1986

Objections Overruled?

What can midwives do if they disagree on professional grounds with a procedure they have been instructed to carry out? Caroline Flint advises them to do their homework, and to have all the evidence at their fingertips to back their argument

I am conscious of anger everywhere. Many women are angry because they feel that their bodies are being taken over, that they have no say in how they will have their babies, where they will have their babies and when they will have their babies.

The anger of women is ignored at our peril - they are the guardians of the future. On their perception of their children's births hinges much of their mental health and well-being and, through them, the mental health and well-being of the community. Their protests seem to be getting shriller. We cannot afford to ignore what the voices are saying.

There is another anger which I am very conscious of at the moment. That is the anger of midwives. I have spoken at several meetings recently and midwives ask me how to cope with having to do things against their will, things which they see as detrimental to women. Many midwives are unconvinced that women should have their membranes ruptured routinely at any particular stage of labour or that routine electronic fetal monitoring actually benefits everybody. They feel confused and treacherous because they feel they are foisting treatments on women which are not helpful and may be downright harmful.

Why are these midwives doing things they don't agree with? Why are they rupturing membranes when they think they should be left intact? Why are they putting fetal scalp electrodes on women who are gravida 3, and 7 cms dilated, in a perfectly normal labour? They are intelligent women. Have they suddenly taken leave of their senses? No, they say, 'it's hospital policy' - as if that explained everything, as if that was the reason night follows day or that falling toast always lands on the buttered side.

What has my reply been to those midwives who have taken me aside and voiced the same deep concerns when talking to me in private places? What about hospital policy?

What if your hospital policy laid down that when a woman comes into this hospital in labour the first midwife to greet her must then jump on her head? Would you do it?

You know that you wouldn't – you know that to have her head jumped on would be detrimental to the woman and very detrimental to your career. You would not comply with that instruction at all.

What is the difference between this instruction, which is obviously ridiculous, and the other instruction which may well be just as ridiculous for the particular woman you are with at this moment?

A professional person has responsibilities and loyalties. Those are (in order):
• To her client
• To her profession
• To her employer

If, in her professional opinion, the midwife feels she is being asked to do something which is detrimental to the welfare of her client, then she not only has a duty to refuse to do it on behalf of her client, she also has a duty to refuse to do it on behalf of her profession.

What if she feels that the pressure is coming from the third in line of responsibility - her employer? One profession cannot change the practice and *modus operandi* of another. I could not issue a decree from *Nursing Times* to architects to say that in future all their plans must be drawn in green ink on recycled paper, even though plans might be much easier to read when written in green ink. If obstetricians also issued this decree to architects, what would happen? Would they instantly take up their green pens as you and I are taking up our amnihooks?

To decline to do what one has been instructed to do needs courage, but above all it needs knowledge. One needs to be able to quote, or even better to produce relevant research on the subject under discussion. You could say, for instance: 'No I haven't ruptured her membranes. I'm very influenced by the work of Dunn[1] who listed the hazards of amniotomy as being, among other things, the loss of isometric uterine contractions (when the pressure is the same throughout) which protects uteroplacental circulation. In addition, Donald[2] describes the assistance of the bulging bag of membranes to the rotation of the fetal head when the baby is in a posterior position. Robson[3] has shown that a woman has a 74 per cent chance of feeling indifferent to her baby if her membranes have been artificially ruptured, while Inch[4] lists many more reasons for and against amniotomy'.

Go to your manager and give her all the up-to-date information on amniotomy. She is as concerned about the future of our profession as you are. She is also as concerned about the health and welfare of women as you are. Go to women such as the local National Childbirth Trust and the local AIMS group. Keep in touch with women you have looked after in childbirth. With knowledge (and with supportive friends) hospital policy, which is irrelevant, can be changed or discounted.

References
1. Dunn, P. (1979). 'Problems associated with fetal monitoring during labour'. In; *Perinatal Medicine.* Sixth European Congress, Vienna. Stuttgart: Georg Thieme, .
2. Donald, I. (1966). *Practical Obstetric Problems.* London: Lloyd–Luke.
3. Robson, K M. (1982). 'Mother-baby relation ship: I feel nothing'. *Nursing Mirror*, Vol.154: pp.24-27.
4. Inch, S. (1982). *Birthrights.* London: Hutchinson.

Reproduced with kind permission from Nursing Times, April 2, 1986

Is it the Unkindest Cut?

*Is delivery by Caesarean section merely another way of having a baby?
Caroline Flint looks at the psychological effects of this procedure on some
mothers and questions its routine use*

I have heard a number of comments in the last month from women searching in anguish for a reason for having had a Caesarean section.

'Caroline', one said, 'I feel that someone has been out and bought any old baby and given it to me.'

'I feel so angry and resentful, was my operation really necessary?'

'It leaves you feeling so weak and drained and then you have a new baby to look after too, you can't help feeling a teeny bit resentful towards the baby.'

'I keep asking myself was it really necessary, did I really need it?'

'I can't get it out of my mind, I keep going over and over it all the time, John is getting really bored with me rabbiting on about it'

Not all women seem to go through this sort of soul-searching, some seem relieved to have a Caesarean, some who have very obvious obstetric problems are perfectly happy about it, but many are obviously anguished - and I don't use the word lightly - about what has happened to them.

When I discuss this with my medical or midwifery colleagues I am aware of a great gap in perception. Most of them see a Caesarean as just another way of having a baby. All these midwives say: 'She shouldn't see it as a failure, it's a success, she's got a live healthy baby.'

I remember how amazed I was when I heard one woman who was holding her very beautiful, live, healthy baby say: 'I feel that nothing good has come out of all this.' She was an intelligent woman - she knew that she had a live, healthy baby, so I didn't negate her feelings by pointing this out to her. But she also knew that she was suffering terribly from an acute sense of loss, a feeling that somehow she hadn't 'made it' as a woman and felt a terrible failure.

In the Tooting maternity unit one in every seven women has a Caesarean section, but this is not uncommonly high for a London hospital - indeed there are several units with a higher percentage. Caesareans are carried out in response to extreme circumstances, but how is it that these circumstances occur more frequently in some units than in others? Could it be something to do with attitudes to childbirth, rather than with the actual physical details of the women concerned?

In 1982, Judith Trowell studied a group of women delivered by emergency Caesarean section and compared them to a group who had a normal vaginal delivery.[1] Her results showed that the Caesarean group encountered more depression, anxiety, doubts about their mothering abilities and indeed their behaviour towards their children was less appropriate to their infants' needs. Altogether, these women had a less happy mothering experience than their sisters who had had normal births. If these Caesareans had been life-saving procedures the cost in relaxed mothering might well have been justified, but if they were carried out just because they took place in St Aloysius' rather than in Nether Wallop maternity unit, does that make the cost justified?

What about the other costs involved in a Caesarean section? In 1976-78 the *Report on Confidential Inquiries into Maternal Deaths* revealed that 90 women had died from the effects associated with Caesarean section. Margaret Ackers was awarded £13,775 last month because she was conscious throughout the Caesarean operation - she has also found a further five women who claim that they went through the same ordeal. In 1982, Samina Sarwar had a Caesarean section. Her baby daughter is now a healthy three year old - the mother has been in a coma ever since she had the operation.

An article about wound infection after Caesarean section[2] (see *Nursing Times* June 5) quoted an infection rate of 5.1 per cent of women who had minor sepsis, 17.49 per cent who had wound inflammation and 1 per cent who had major sepsis in which the integrity of the wound was threatened. Think of the cost in terms of human suffering, the amount of antibiotics with their associated cost - the amount of anxiety and worry about wounds breaking down, the number of extra days spent in hospital.

A Caesarean section is a major abdominal operation - women feel weak for months afterwards, they have problems picking up their baby and they feel anxious and inadequate as mothers. It is not just another way of having a baby, it is a dangerous and risky and mutilating procedure and its sequelae are far-reaching and momentous. It can be a life-saving operation, and it can be the best way of delivery some babies, but let us never lose sight of its other costs which for some women may be too high a price to pay if the only reason for it is the obstetricians' peace of mind. Perhaps we need to get away from the philosophy that it's alright to interfere but it's not alright to do nothing and allow nature to take its course. We should only interfere when we can definitely improve on nature - and that isn't too often.

References
1. Trowell, J. (1982). 'Possible effects of emergency Caesarean section on the mother-child relationship.' *Early Human Develop ment*, 7: pp. 41-51
2. Moir-Bussy, B., Hutton, R., Thompson, J. (1985). 'Wound infection after Caesarean section.' *Journal of Infection Control Nursing. Nursing Times*; Vol. 81: 23, pp.13-14.

Reproduced with kind permission from Nursing Times, July 3 1985

Fact–finding Mission

Does it matter how many episiotomies, inductions or Caesarean sections are performed in your delivery unit? Caroline Flint argues that midwives can easily carry out this type of research locally, and that this could ultimately affect obstetric practice

What is really happening to the women midwives are looking after? What affects them? What affects their care? Is the care we are giving the most appropriate? The most needed or the most desired?

Is midwifery care based on the wishes of each individual woman, or is it based on a scientific and reasonable assessment of the needs of this particular woman, her baby and her partner? Or does her outcome depend on the time of day, the day of the week, or even on who is on duty?

Midwives are in a unique position to find out the answers to hundreds of questions affecting women. There is a great deal of research they can do easily, cheaply, with little effort and which may influence midwifery and obstetric practice and what happens to women.

Midwives are there – there in the antenatal clinic, in the labour ward, in the postnatal ward and in the community. Midwives actually see what is happening and they have a special opportunity to report it to their colleagues.

There are several questions worth asking. For example, does the Caesarean section rate in your delivery suite go up every Tuesday evening because a certain doctor is on duty? Is this useful or helpful to the women? Could you look back in the birth register and work out the numbers of Caesarean sections performed each day and point out how it increases when Dr X is on duty? Perhaps the birth register will show that in fact the Caesarean section rate on Tuesday evenings is no different from any other day. Perhaps

they occur even less, and that it is your basic antipathy to Dr X which brought you to your original conclusion – whatever result you come up with you can't fail.

If you show that Dr X does more Caesareans than average and if you alert him to this fact, perhaps he will be more circumspect in his practice in the future. This will help him and will be beneficial to the women coming to your hospital.

If you show that Dr X does less than or the same proportion of Caesareans as the average it is a chance for you to revise your opinion of Dr X.

The birth register is the easiest of all research tools, enabling you to do research with no extra equipment, no searching for notes, no literature searches and no expense. Kept on every labour ward, the birth register can answer so many questions and those answers can make such a difference to the way women are treated in a unit.

Traditionally, we have thought that women aged under 18 and over 35 are at a higher risk during pregnancy than those who are between those ages. But is this still true? Can you find out what birth outcomes women in these two categories have in your unit? Will it benefit anyone if you do?

If you find out that these women fare exactly the same as anyone else then probably they will be deemed suitable for a midwife's care during more of their pregnancy and labour. But if you find out that these women fare worse than other women, you have accentuated the known body of knowledge and your work will ensure that these women have more medical care than they otherwise would.

How many episiotomies are carried out in your unit? Valerie Wilkerson found that one midwife in her unit performed episiotomies on 92.8 per cent of women having a first baby, while another midwife carried out this procedure on only 12.5 per cent of these women.[1] Is this what happens in your unit? Does the episiotomy depend on the midwife supervising the delivery rather than on fetal distress, old scar tissue or an impending large tear?

What proportion of women in your unit are induced? Is it ten per cent or 45 per cent? Does it matter whether they are induced or not? Sheila Kitzinger, in her report to the DHSS in 1975 and 1978 quotes a higher rate of instrumental deliveries in women having induced births, higher levels of analgesia, babies with more respiratory depression and more babies admitted to the special care baby unit[2].

Again, if you proved this to be wrong in your unit you would have scotched a myth.

If you proved it to be correct you would have alerted your obstetric colleagues to the hazards of being induced in your unit and you would have helped countless women to avoid unnecessary intervention. Read these paragraphs again but for *induction* substitute *acceleration.*

As midwives we have a duty to the women and families in our care to ascertain that they are having the care that is most appropriate and desirable for them. As we become more aware of quality control we shall be providing figures to our general managers and ultimately to our clients, with information on what they can expect in our unit compared with St Nibs down the road. If midwives can be one jump ahead here we shall be doing mothers and their families a good turn. So come on – get cracking!

References

Wilkerson, V. (1984). 'The use of episiotomy in normal delivery.' *Midwives Chronicle and Nursing Notes* April, pp.106-110.

Kitzinger, S. (1978). *Some Mothers' Experiences of Induced Labour.* London: The National Childbirth Trust.

Reproduced with kind permission from Nursing Times, May 22 1985

Midwives and Breastfeeding

Breastfeeding is a very private and personal experience, says Caroline Flint.
Midwives should be enablers rather than helpers

'The two lie close in each other's arms, dark eyes gazing into dark eyes, breaths soft and panting as the erect, hot tissue searches for the soft, most, open orifice.'

A description of lovemaking? It could be just that, but what if one of the two is only six days' old, or six weeks, or six hours? Then it is, of course, a description of breastfeeding. The similarity between the two very intimate experiences is not only in the fact that the nipple is composed of erectile tissue and that the baby's mouth is open and moist, but that the breastfeeding women releases oxytocin from the posterior lobe of the pituitary gland just as she does when she is in labour and when she is making love.

Just like lovemaking, breastfeeding is described as 'natural' but it is interesting to note that in 1980 only 12 per cent of women were feeding their babies 'naturally' by the time their babies were nine months' old, and that by four months' old (the DHSS recommended length of breastfeeding) only 26 per cent of mothers were 'naturally' feeding their babies.[1]

What is the point of comparing breastfeeding to lovemaking? We all know that midwives are trying to encourage breastfeeding, and that indeed the prevalence of breastfeeding of four-month-old babies has increased from 13 per cent in 1975 to 26 per cent in 1980[1]. Very few women going through the antenatal system miss out on having their breasts examined; many of them have advice on expressing colostrum, wearing supporting bras, rolling nipples, washing nipples, creaming or oiling nipples. Midwives all over the country are bent over nipples examining, advising and educating.

Once the baby is born, midwives again see their role as a provider of 'help' and 'education' for the breastfeeding mother. The newborn baby is expected to 'latch on' within the first hour following birth and although I applaud the time span, I question the way the 'latching on' is accomplished. During the following days the baby is put to the breast frequently and, thankfully, nearly all hospitals now practise real demand feeding, that is, feeding whenever the baby wants. But what else does the baby receive in the hospital? Are we really helping women when they are breastfeeding. Could we be perhaps termed as obstructive, or unhelpful?

We should look at breastfeeding as an intimate, physical experience between two people. Ask any mother and she will tell you that each of her children were different when breastfeeding. 'Johnny was so easy'; 'Mary wasn't interested for days, and when she did suck, she sucked at a funny angle and made my nipple sore. I evolved a technique of feeding her lying down and then it didn't hurt'; 'Justin stayed on the breast for hours at a time. Each time he dropped off to sleep I'd try to take him off, and then he began sucking furiously again'.

Is it the same experience with each sexual partner a person has? Does every human being in the land make love in the same way? I suggest not. Likewise, it would seem rational that every baby in the land should breastfeed slightly differently and that the feeding of each baby is just that - *the feeding of this baby* - not the feeding of any baby.

Think about the first experience of breastfeeding; the woman lying or sitting on the delivery table, the midwife 'helping' by holding the baby's head in one hand and the woman's breast in the other. Imagine if the first experience of lovemaking were the same, with an 'expert' at the side of the bed organising the young man and the young woman, pushing them into the 'right' position, compering the whole event: 'Now, John come a little to the right, that's right, Jane, move your leg here, now John ...' Describing this ridiculous scene makes me laugh, but we do it all the time when a woman is starting to breastfeed. How useful is this sort of 'help'? Would it perhaps be more useful, and indeed more of a boost to a women's confidence, if we left her and her baby (with her partner) and said, as we left to make the tea and write up our notes, 'He looks as if he'd like to have a feed. Put him to the breast while I'm away'. The parents left to get their baby onto the breast can usually achieve this without any problems, and when the midwife returns, the baby has often been suckling for 20 minutes and the proud parents are beaming with pleasure because 'they did it'.

The greatest need of a mother is confidence in herself. We can affect her level of confidence by the sort of support we give her during labour, by the amount and sort of analgesia she (and therefore the baby) receives. A baby who has received little or no analgesia (or whose mother has had an epidural) is likely to be more alert and interested in breastfeeding during the first few hours and days than the baby who has received large quantities of analgesics during labour.

A newborn baby's head is very sensitive, and if someone holds it, it will instinctively root towards the hand, hence the 'struggle' noted when midwives hold the baby's head and clamp it to the mother's breast.

So, I am suggesting that::
• breastfeeding is an intimate, physical partnership which needs to be carried out (initially) in private by the two people concerned
• the role of the midwife is not a physical or practical role but rather that of a 'cheer leader': 'Aren't you doing well?' 'Doesn't he enjoy it?' 'You feed your baby beautifully'.
• the baby - this baby - should control the feeding, when, how long, how much.
• everything that could reduce a woman's confidence in her ability to feed her baby should be moved - bottles of water or formula.
• scales should not be strategically placed in the postnatal ward, for these also reduce a woman's confidence. Any midwife worthy of the name can tell if a baby is thriving.

Finally, I am suggesting that we need to evaluate what we are doing. Can we leave women alone to get on with breastfeeding and just help them with encouraging words? Or is it better for us to be handling women's breasts (could this be so embarrassing for the woman that it could impede the release of oxytocin) and 'fixing' the baby to the breast? Are we helping women to breastfeed? Or are we hindering with excessive interference?

We shall only know when someone does a randomized controlled trial - could that be you?

Reference
Office of Population Censuses and Surveys (1982). *Infant Feeding*. London.

Further Reading
Messenger, M. (1982). *The Breastfeeding Book*. Century Publishing Ltd.
Stanway, P.A. (1978). *Breast is Best*. London: Pan Books.
Kitzinger, S. (1979). The *Experience of Breastfeeding*. Harmondsworth: Penguin Books.
La Leche League Book (1971). *The Womanly Art of Breastfeeding*.

Reproduced with kind permission from Nursing Times, April 11, 1984

Cosiness in the Delivery Suite

Labour wards should be comfortable, home-like places, says Caroline Flint.
Here she makes some suggestions on how to improve them

Throughout the country we are trying to 'humanize' our labour wards. We are trying to make them more comfortable, more relaxed, cosier and more like home.

I lay in bed this morning and tried to think of what the essence of a bedroom is. I looked around my own familiar bedroom and in my imagination tried to transport myself to a delivery room in our hospital, and then I compared the difference.

First, and probably most importantly, no strangers ever come into my bedroom. The door never flies open letting a stranger in, either to borrow some equipment or to check me over or to discuss anything with my companion. People only enter my bedroom by invitation' even my children knock and wait for permission before coming in to look for their socks in the airing cupboard, or to ask for their dinner money.

I thought about being in a delivery room/my bedroom and being in labour and realised that if I transferred my bedroom to the labour ward I'd want to be able to bolt or lock the door to stop strangers from walking in especially if I were undressing, having a vaginal examination, having my abdomen palpated, using a bedpan or being emotional and was being comforted by a midwife, companion or husband.

The lack of privacy in labour wards, even in the most enlightened of hospitals, came over very strongly recently. We had a woman in labour and her contractions were going off; we suggested that her husband should stimulate her nipples and that we would leave them in private for 15 minutes.[1]

Because our delivery rooms have no way of being locked, the student midwife and I had to take turns in 'standing guard' outside the room so that the couple were not disturbed.

The other invasion of privacy in most delivery wards are the grills in the doors, similar to the peepholes in prison cells. Most enlightened hospitals have covered their 'spy-holes' with paper or had them removed, but it is worth imagining the effect that these 'spy-holes' would have on you if there were one in your own bedroom door and when you looked up there was a pair of strange eyes looking at you. Hardly conducive to the relaxed release of oxytocin by a labouring woman.

The most important feature in most bedrooms is the bed. I imagined the bed in my transported bedroom/delivery room. The essence of my bed is that it is comfortable, I can lie in it for eight, 10, or even 12 hours with comfort. When I had 'flu two months ago I lay in bed for four days and suffered no stiffness, no pressure sores, no discomfort. The other great pleasure of my bed is that it is cosy, when I stretch out there is the warm and reassuring presence of my beloved husband. Double beds are perhaps the most companionable places ever designed and for people who have been sharing their lives with a partner this is perhaps the greatest deprivation of all when they come into hospital.

I remember, when I was a nurse working at night in a gynaecological ward, I heard little sobs coming from the far end of the ward, and when I went to investigate I found a woman in tears, who said, 'I put my hand

57

out to find him, and he wasn't there'. Even as a young nurse with no experience of sharing a bed it moved me to tears.

Other memories come flooding back. After our first baby was born at home, one of the most magical experiences for both of us was the new family, snuggling down in bed together with arms around each other listening to baby Matthew snuffling and sucking his fist. I often think of that when fathers who have just gone through the same experience, say goodbye to their new baby and their partner who lies pristinely in her single bed in the postnatal ward.

Another memory is very recent. Two weeks ago when a couple had given birth to a stillborn baby, like all caring hospitals nowadays, the husband was allowed - even encouraged - to stay to support and share their grief together. When I knocked and came into their bedroom the morning after their tragedy, the wife was already awake. Lying at the end of her bed on one of the hospital's little portable beds was her husband, sleeping soundly. I asked her how she had slept and she said wistfully, 'I really missed Derek; he seemed so far away. We tried with both of us lying in the bed, but it was too precarious.' My heart went out to her, this grieving woman who only wanted someone's arms around her. If only she had been in a double bed this would have happened without thought or effort.

Another memory is of a couple whose baby I had delivered who had a breathing problem. The baby was in the special care baby unit. The mother, now past her 10 days, was staying in the mother's bedroom in the SCBU. I knocked on the door, timidly, I knew that the news was not good. When I was invited in, a touching scene was revealed. Mother and father had managed to snuggle together on the narrow bed in order to cuddle and comfort each other.

In many labour wards great efforts are being made with wallpaper, pictures and pretty bedspreads. If the bedspreads are going on the hard platforms which are more reminiscent of an ironing board than a bed,

then is there really any point? I often feel that we midwives and our colleagues should all spend one night's 'sleep' on one of our delivery 'beds' and see how we feel in the morning. I imagine we should all feel stiff, bruised and uncomfortable.

Many hospitals have of course recognized the inadequacies of the conventional delivery bed and they are spending several thousands of pounds on highly sophisticated 'birthing beds' or 'birthing chairs' which turn into beds complete with lithotomy poles at the touch of a switch. In frustration, the Association of Radical Midwives, having realized that most women are still giving birth on these hard platforms, has designed a cheap birthing bar which will slot into the holes where the lithotomy poles go, so that women will have more opportunity to move around during labour even when confined to the bed.

At our own hospital we are blessed with soft mats which we put on the floor and cover with a clean sheet so that women can crawl, squat or flop as they please. We also have wonderful plastic-covered beanbags which they lie back in to deliver, or lean against to deliver on all fours. We keep the conventional delivery beds just outside the door, readily available if complications occur and we need to put the woman into the lithotomy position. All the beds are on wheels so it only takes a second to bring them into the delivery room.

My suggestions for 'humanizing' the labour ward are simple and above all cheap. Labour wards will only become 'cosy' when we buy double beds so that during labour and after the birth, a couple can cuddle and support each other. The cost of a double bed is only £400 at the most; a lock or bolt only costs a couple of pounds but think of the difference they would both make!

Reference
1. Lenke, R.R., Nemes, J.M. (1984). 'Use of nipple stimulation to obtain contraction stress test.' *American Journal of Obtetrics and Gynaecology*; Vol. 63: No 3.

Reproduced with kind permission from Nursing Times, June 13, 1984

Postpartum Haemorrhage at Home

Jane was keen to have a home birth, and in spite of her GPs opposition, Stefan was born according to plan. But immediately after the birth Jane began to haemorrhage. Caroline Flint explains how she coped

Harry and Jane decided to have their baby at home 14 days before he was due. Originally they had tried for a domino delivery but had been discouraged because of Jane's 'advanced years' (37) and because it was her first pregnancy.

What they had expected in a domino (domiciliary in-and-out) delivery was that Jane would be cared for at home in the early part of her labour, and the same midwife would deliver her in hospital and take her home again shortly afterwards. However, in the area in which Jane and Harry lived, the reality meant being attended by any one of 14 midwives, most of whom they would not know, and being assessed in the labour ward, again by an unknown midwife.

As her pregnancy progressed, it became increasingly important to Jane that she knew who was going to deliver her and, co-incidentally, she became increasingly attracted to a home birth. It was important to her not to be separated from Harry in the first few days of their child's life and she was fairly strong in her wish to have as little medical intervention as possible. She thought this might be difficult to avoid in hospital.

Jane had also discovered that she might have to stay in hospital longer than the six hours she was prepared to after the baby's birth because of difficulties in getting an ambulance to take her home, and a paediatrician to discharge her baby to the care of the community midwife. Often, women waited for several hours because the paediatrician was busy with ill babies. So she decided to have her baby at home with independent midwives. When my partner, Lorna, and I went to book Jane and Harry we studied her co-operation card and discovered that her pregnancy had progressed normally except for an episode of high blood pressure (130/85mmHg) at 36 weeks, compared with Jane's booking blood pressure of 100/60mmHg. But at 37 weeks it had returned to 120/80mmHg.

Jane was pregnant for the first time at 37, she was 5ft 5in. (1.5m) tall and had a shoe size of five with normal bone formation of both hands and feet. Her blood group was Rhesus positive and her haemoglobin at 37 weeks was 11.8g/dl.

Lorna and I took a full and detailed history of Jane's previous health, her menstrual history, Harry's health and how they had both been born and fed. We asked about their families and discussed the possibility of having someone to help for the first fortnight after the birth while Jane and Harry were tied up with the new baby.

Lorna and I pointed out the two risks in home birth, haemorrhage and a baby needing resuscitation. In the event of haemorrhage we carry Syntometrine and Haemacel plus an intravenous giving set. If the baby needs resuscitation we carry suckers, bag and mask and oxygen. It is ironic that we tell women the dangers of home birth when they are not told the dangers inherent in opting for a hospital birth.

We visited Jane and Harry three times in the 13 days before Jane went into labour. This was to do antenatal checks but mainly to get to know them and to enable them to get to know us and to make sure that they had obtained everything on our list ready for their birth.

The day we booked Jane and Harry, I wrote to the supervisor of midwives to take out an intention to practise and to inform her that we had booked Jane for a home birth. I also told her that I had written to Jane's GP and informed him that if he would like to be involved, I should be very pleased, but that if he did not I would immediately contact the obstetric unit if any illness or abnormality occurred in either mother or baby.

The day after they had booked with us, Jane and Harry went to see their GP for a routine antenatal check and to tell him that they had decided to have their baby at home. Both were somewhat upset by the experience, not because of the GP's attitude that they were taking an enormous risk but because of the emotiveness of the encounter; it took a good deal of restraint on their part not to respond to the GP's evident anger and they felt a little more objectivity would have been in order.

Jane and Harry questioned us about the dangers of having a baby at Jane's age. We pointed out the increased risk of high blood pressure but as Jane's blood pressure was 100/50mmHg when we visited her this did not seem to be a cause for immediate anxiety!

Meanwhile, I had had a telephone call from the GP who had contacted the Medical Defence Union who had told him that he was still responsible for the birth even though he had declined to be there, and that he had better strike her off his list in order to opt out of the involvement. I had a quick consultation with local legal opinion and telephoned him back to point out that if I had assured him that I would not call him during the birth, he could not be accused of negligence in a birth that he knew nothing about.

At 5.00 am the next day Jane went into labour. She had woken to pass urine and her contractions had started half-an-hour later. She called me at 6.35 am and I arrived at 7.10 am to have a cup of tea with Harry and Jane

(the first of many) and noticed that Jane was relaxing well through her contractions leaning on the kitchen work surface. I took her temperature and pulse, which were normal, and her blood pressure which was 90/50mmHg. The baby was in a cephalic presentation with his head engaged, left occipito-lateral, and his heart was beating regularly at 124/min.

On vaginal examination, Jane's cervix was 2-3 cm dilated and fully effaced, the position was central to posterior. The baby's head was 1 cm above the ischial spines and Jane was having strong but short contractions every five minutes.

We settled down for the labour and it progressed smoothly. Jane liked having her back massaged during contractions. She spent time in the bath, leaning forwards on a bean bag, leaning forward on the stairs, on all fours and rocking to and fro. During labour she had ketones in her urine which we counteracted with fruit teas containing honey. Jane was in good spirits throughout her labour while having a good grumble about the pain. She carried on having fairly short contractions every four minutes but they appeared to be fairly effective.

She maintained an empty bladder and at 6.25 pm her membranes ruptured with streaks of meconium staining the liquor. On vaginal examination Jane was fully dilated, the baby's heart was excellent, between 128 and 144/min, so we were not concerned about the baby's condition. Lorna and I decided that the best position for Jane to deliver would be either standing or on hands-and-knees so that the baby's mouth could be sucked out really effectively before the birth of the chest. Jane delivered on all fours and we sucked out Stefan's mouth, throat and nose very thoroughly as this position allows for really efficient aspiration. This position also encourages any mucous to flow out of the baby's mouth and nose. Stefan arrived at 7.27 pm and his Apgar score was 9 (because he was slightly blue), 10 at 5 minutes and 10 at 10 minutes. He emerged looking glad to be here.

We sucked him out again when the whole of his body had been delivered and found the aspirate mucoid and Stefan's chest sounded completely clear. Jane sat on my bedpan cuddling Stefan. Harry thrilled at the birth, took photos and we chatted and exclaimed with pleasure at what had taken place and waited for the contraction heralding the placenta. I looked into the bedpan and thought that the placenta had arrived already because there was something dark red and large in the pan. It was then that I realized that Jane was bleeding. The Syntometrine was already drawn up and we gave this to Jane immediately and felt her uterus which was contracted.

I then delivered the placenta by controlled cord traction while Harry held the baby and Lorna, my partner, supported Jane as she sat on the bedpan. Once the placenta was delivered we transferred Jane to bed – she felt extremely weak and shaky, her pulse was 94 and her blood pressure 120/90mmHg. She looked horribly pale and just wanted to lie down. Her uterus was well contracted but from looking at the bedpan she had obviously lost a great deal of blood. Jane's blood pressure and pulse remained within normal limits but all she wanted to do was lie still and rest.

The baby was safe with Harry who was chatting to him and keeping him warm in his arms but what about Jane? Here she was looking shocked and pale, having lost one litre of blood. The placenta was complete but it had obviously been embedded in the lower segment of the uterus and the uterus had bled because the lower segment does not contract as well as the upper segment.

I looked at Jane, she looked pale and weak but had stopped bleeding once the placenta was delivered. I felt weak myself and wondered why I was here in a house and not in a nice warm hospital with nice warm doctors all around me! The emergency was past, an intravenous infusion with Haemacel was not indicated nor was transfer to hospital because nothing could be done there that

couldn't be done at home. Jane's blood would be taken for haemoglobin estimation and if she needed transfusing afterwards she would be transfused, but what about Midwives' Rules? 'In any case where there is an emergency or a deviation from norm in the health of a mother or baby a midwife shall call to her assistance a registered medical practitioner.'

It seemed pointless to phone the hospital to explain that we had had a postpartum haemorrhage in the community and had treated it at home and were not going to come in. What about the GP? We could hardly telephone him. I fretted about this as I sutured Jane's second degree tear.

Afterwards I discussed my dilemma with the supervisor of midwives, 'You should have rung me of course ,' she said, 'There's a supervisor of midwives on call at all times, we could have made reassuring noises down the telephone and you would have been fulfilling the duties laid down in the Rules.' I realized how much better I would have felt had I done that. She also suggested sitting women on an incontinence pad rather than a bedpan which tends to hide the amount of blood been lost.

We visited Jane three times a day for the first three days as she seemed so weak and looked so pale. We made sure that she was taking extra iron in the form of iron tablets, a herbal iron preparation, yeast tablets, liver, molasses, parsley, watercress, stout and raisins. We tended baby Stefan, and Jane used a bedpan for passing urine. She was able to go to the bath the day after Stefan's birth, with assistance, although we offered her a bed-bath because she seemed shaky. She was, however, at pains to reassure everyone that she looked far worse than she felt.

Jane's haemoglobin the day after the birth was 9.8g/dl which did not indicate the need for a blood transfusion. We encouraged her to move her feet and legs in order to avoid a deep vein thrombosis. I informed Jane's GP the day after the delivery and he visited and examined Stefan the following day. I told him

Jane's haemoglobin and when, on the ninth day, her haemoglobin was 8.8g/dl, I rang him again to tell him this result. He pointed out that it was likely that the original specimen was inaccurate as the level of leucocytes, phagocytes, lymphocytes, and fibrinogen rises at the beginning of labour and the blood becomes more concentrated during labour because the woman becomes slightly dehydrated.

The specimen I took initially was probably concentrated and Jane's haemoglobin had actually been much lower.

The GP suggested taking another specimen the following day and seeing whether Jane's haemoglobin had increased at all and asking for a reticulocyte count which would show whether she was actually making new red blood cells for herself. This I did; the haemoglobin was 9.0g/dl and the reticulocytes 4.4/100 RBC's (normal range 0.2 - 2.0/100 RBC's), showing that Jane was indeed making new red blood cells as fast as her body could.

Stefan thrived, he fed frequently and with enthusiasm and despite Jane's anaemic state he went from 8lb 11oz (3.94kg) at birth to 9lb 7oz (4.28kg) on day six and to 12lb (5.44kg) when we discharged him and his mother at 28 days. At six weeks Jane's haemoglobin was 13.0 g/dl and her reticulocyte count was 0.8 per cent , she seemed so well and had adapted well to life as a mother and was enjoying her lovely son. Harry clearly adored Stefan and spent many happy hours cooing at him and discussing the problems of the world with him, at the same time grumbling about how much time he took up!

Reproduced with kind permission from Nursing Times, Vol. 84, No. 3 January 20 1988

Skills Behind the Scenes

The skills and knowledge exclusive to midwives can mean the difference between a mechanized birth and a normal, natural delivery. Caroline Flint describes the unique contribution of midwives to success in pregnancy and labour

You can't get a diploma by sitting and waiting patiently. You can't get a degree for talking someone through a stressful and painful experience in a supportive way. You can't get a doctorate for knowing in your bones that something isn't quite right. And so it is that one of the greatest problems for midwives is that their knowledge and skills are often indefinable, instinctive, and sometimes not easy to describe.

Frequently, they don't realize that they've got knowledge at all and if they do they don't think of it as anything special. They do not even realize that it could make all the difference for a woman between having a normal, unmedicated birth, feeling incredibly clever and proud of herself or having a birth complicated by analgesics, possibly an instrumental delivery and feeling that she had no part in the birth of her baby.

Because midwives are unaware of their value and worth neither is anyone else. Midwives recognize the special skills and knowledge of the obstetrician: the ability to deliver by forceps; the surgical skills involved in doing a Caesarean section; the ability to put up intravenous drips or to carry out fetal blood sampling and to interpret the results.

Both obstetricians and midwives usually recognize the areas of skill in which both overlap: Midwives' ability to do vaginal examinations; to ascertain the position of the baby *in utero* ; to read fetal heart tracings; to suture perineums, resuscitate babies; to know about the progress of labour and deviations from the normal and similarly with pregnancy and the puerperium.

In an interesting paper in the *British Journal of Obstetrics and Gynaecology* (1983, p.123) Michael Klein points out that women who were cared for in their own homes in early labour by community midwives enjoyed a number of advantages over a comparable group who did not have the benefit of a community midwife. Although they were generally in labour for longer, they spent comparatively less time in the labour ward, had fewer epidurals, received less pethidine, fewer forceps deliveries, had babies with higher Apgar scores and a higher number who needed no intubation.

But equally important are the knowledge and skills that are exclusive to the midwife.

For example, waiting is perhaps the most important skill for anyone involved in the often slow process of birth. It is the skill that has denigrated since the advent of active management of labour, but I suggest that there is a much needed place for it and that it is the midwives who are able to provide it.

Women in the antenatal period really appreciate a health professional who shows real interest in her as a person. Midwives don't find this difficult and often their special skills ensure that their antenatal consultations are warm and caring and much appreciated by their clients.

Again, by concentrating on the normality of childbirth when a woman is in highly suggestible state it wouldn't seem too far fetched to suggest that perhaps the midwife ensures normality of outcome. This was a point which was recognized by the midwives' boards before their demise in their excellent booklet, *The Role of the Midwife*[1] which suggested; ' Perhaps one of the main threats to the execution of the midwife's role is the practical application of the philosophy that childbirth is normal only in retrospect'.

Despite the increased use of episiotomy over the past decade many midwives are still able to deliver with an intact perineum or minimal trauma and since the research conducted by midwife Jennifer Sleep[2] many midwives are re-learning this skill.

Another skill exclusive to midwives is the hostess role. It is easy for the midwife to offer the newly-admitted labouring woman and her partner a cup of tea and for her to provide light refreshments throughout labour and after. This not only emphasizes the normality of labour but also helps to avoid ketosis.[3]

Midwives also have the patience and the interest to wait patiently but all the time encouraging the woman, while she and her baby get breastfeeding organized.

An interest in and knowledge of pelvic floors and perineums again are the province of the midwife. The list is very long but these skills have something in common – they are all quiet skills, skills for which one can receive no paper qualification, skills which are unassuming, for which it would be difficult to get a prize. But nevertheless we mustn't underestimate them – for the women we care for, for the women we are with, these skills are of paramount importance.

References
1. Central Midwives Board for Scotland, Northern Ireland Council for Nurses and Midwives, An Bord Altranais, Central Midwives Board. *The role of the Midwife*
2. Sleep, J. (1984). 'Episiotomy in normal delivery'. *Nursing Times* 80:47; pp. 29-30; 48, 51-54.
3. Haire, D. (1972). *The Cultural Warping of Childbirth* London: International Childbirth Education Association.

Reproduced with kind permission from Nursing Times, March 6 1985

Rules, Laws, Autonomy and Justice

This section deals with the marriage between midwifery and the law. It is a relationship personified within the Flint household. Giles Flint is a lawyer and his knowledge has been a resource Caroline has made effective use of on many occasions. Another lawyer friendly to midwifery is Ronald Briggs, who after writing a letter to *The Times* deploring the treatment of Jilly Rosser, was contacted by Caroline, became persuaded of the merits of the case for a new Midwives Act and became instrumental in drawing up the draft act mentioned in 'Why Do Midwives want a new Act?'. Such networking can prove invaluable and lead to not very obvious but worthwhile courses of action, such as the Association of Radical Midwives (ARM) petitioning of the Lord Chancellor regarding the Professional Conduct Rules of the United Kingdom Central Council for Nursing, Midwifery and Health Visiting (UKCC), ('Juno Lucina, March 1989'). The Professional Conduct machinery has subsequently been reformed in line with many of the suggestions put forward by ARM. As many of these articles make clear, Caroline believes that knowing the system, or knowing someone who does, is essential for midwives' empowerment

That belief also leads Caroline to acquire and assiduously comment on any report or proposal that may be relevant to midwifery. The purpose of a number of these articles is to bring such reports to the attention of midwives and to try to encourage them to read and respond to them ('Getting it Right for Mother and Baby', 'A Mother's Birthright' and 'Rules for Midwives'). It may have been a slight exaggeration to suggest that 'midwives are meeting throughout the country to discuss the proposed rules sent out for consultation' ('Rules for Midwives') but Caroline has always made sure that any group of midwives that she has anything to do with get their two penny worth of comments sent in. As the branch secretary or chairperson of the Southern Thames Branch of the RCM for 15 years, she has socialized many dozens of midwives into this somewhat unusual habit.

Caroline's articles on the Short Report ('Getting it Right for Mother and Baby') and Maternity Care in Action Part 2 ('A Mother's Birthright') contain spirited defences of home birth. Her conviction that the crude statistics did not do justice to homebirth in terms of safety has been confirmed by the work of Marjorie Tew (1990). Caroline had all three of her children at home long before she qualified as a midwife (she did the old Part I immediately before her marriage and did not return to nursing or midwifery for 12 years). These extremely happy experiences, particularly the birth of her eldest child, have underpinned her beliefs and practice and made her active in the defence and promotion of homebirth. This zeal, shared by a growing minority remains largely incomprehensible to most of those with no first-hand experience of modern homebirth. Furthermore, homebirth has come to symbolize a model of childbirth that is at odds with the technical model associated with hospitalized birth. This much analysed and discussed dichotomy is at the root of many of the issues raised in the articles in this section, namely those which pertain to the Supervision of Midwives.

During the 1980s a growing number of midwives faced disciplinary action and even suspension from practice. Many of these midwives were 'radical' midwives and/or committed to homebirth and/or in independent practice. A large proportion also happened to be Caroline's personal friends and she used her regular columns in the professional press to argue in their defence and to expose the mess that too many midwifery managers were making of Supervision. The most drawn out case was that of Jilly Rosser for whom there was no 'guide, counsellor and friend' following a client's postnatal collapse at home. Her interrogation by the Professional Conduct Committee of the UKCC was the final nail in the coffin of many midwives' waning belief in the ability of the profession to deal with its members fairly.

'The Golden Thread', written for the Association of Radical Midwives Magazine, was penned in response to the predicament Caroline found herself in as a result of 'Postpartum Haemorrhage at Home' (see Section Three). She was the most fed up with midwifery that she has probably ever been. The remaining articles on the Supervision of midwifery and professional disciplinary procedures have two overriding messages: midwifery supervision has presupposed an outmoded model of midwifery and has failed to adapt to different ways of delivering care and the definitions of normality on which the Midwives Rules and Code of Practice depend are narrow and restricting. Whilst some progress may have been made with the first, the second issue remains one of the most crucial for midwives and women.

Three articles in this section argue the case for a new Midwives Act. The campaign for new and separate legislation arose directly from the decision, in 1989, of the English National Board for Nursing, Midwifery and Health Visiting in favour of generic education officers (though discontent with the statutory framework had been brewing for some time). Caroline was active in the Midwives Legislation Group which successfully raised awareness of the issues not only in midwifery but also amongst doctors and lay groups. The drive for a new act failed however to galvanize the essential support of the Royal College of Midwives. The Commission mentioned in 'Why do Midwives want a New Act? effectively shackled the College to a short-term pragmatism instead of a long-term strategy. In 1994, this pragmatism gained the upper hand when the RCM conference voted against campaigning for a new midwives act, thereby overturning the motion passed in 1990. Meanwhile the Midwives Legislation Group watches and waits.

Reference
Tew, M. (1990). *Safer Childbirth? A Critical History of Maternity Care.* London: Chapman and Hall.

A Midwife's Nightmare

In what circumstances can a midwife be suspended from practice? Caroline Flint describes one midwife's nightmare

I have just arrived back from the International Confederation of Midwives in the Hague - for the past week I have been talking to and meeting midwives from all over the world; from Spain and Malta, Holland, Sweden, France, Africa, Asia, Iceland, Canada and the United States. I have met midwives practising illegally and midwives protected by law. I have been moved by the universality of our problems, the increasing medical takeover of birth throughout the world with its resultant increase in surgery for women having babies, and the universal struggle midwives are having because nursing organisations are trying to annexe them.

I have felt part of a great sisterhood of dedicated women trying to improve childbirth for women, to make it safer and happier, to promote the health of women throughout the world - I have felt proud to be a midwife and I have felt very proud to be an English midwife, protected by our Rules and our Code of Practice.

I felt happy and strong when I walked into my kitchen - I'd only been away for a week but in that week I had grown in knowledge, experience and understanding of midwifery in other countries. England isn't perfect, but it's not so bad really, it's a good place to be a midwife compared to many places - and then the phone rang.

It was my friend Jilly, an independent midwife. 'Caroline, I've been suspended from practice.' I couldn't bear to take it in - the nightmare was starting again.

'Why?'

'Because I took a woman to hospital in private car instead of an ambulance as the nearest hospital was five minutes away and if I had called the obstetric flying squad it would have taken 20 minutes from leaving the hospital, much less getting ready to leave.'

'Jilly, are sure that you have been suspended from practice? How do you know?'

'The supervisor of midwives told me that she was suspending me from practice and she wrote it in a letter.'

'Jilly, a supervisor of midwives cannot suspend you from practice - only the Local Supervising Authority can do that. Have you had a letter from the English National Board telling you that they are investigating a case against you and asking you to give your side of the story?'

'No', said Jilly.

'Then you have not been suspended legally and the whole thing is nullified.'

According to the Midwives' Rules a midwife may be suspended from practice if a case against her has been reported for investigation to a board - the only way a midwife can be suspended immediately, as Jilly had been, was if she was likely to spread infection.

I suggested that Jilly should ignore the 'suspension' and carry on practising, having told the supervisor why she was ignoring it. Easy enough to say, but as all midwives do in this situation, Jilly felt vulnerable and intimidated. She also couldn't contact the supervisor who was away on holiday and there was no other supervisor available in the health authority. The story was getting worse and worse - there should be a supervisor available at all times to be contacted by midwives in the area.

The safety of every midwife's practice is overseen by the Local Supervising Authority - this body is usually referred to as the LSA and in practice it is invariably the regional health authority. It has the power to suspend a midwife from practice if she is the source of infection, if a case against her has been put before the investigating committee, the professional conduct committee or the health committee of the national boards. Only when a case against her has been brought may the LSA suspend a midwife and the midwife will always know if a case against her has gone to the board because she will always be notified by letter and asked to give her side of the case.

To stem the tide of 'suspensions' carried out by supervisors of midwives last year the UKCC issued a circular (PC/86/03) which stated, 'It should be noted that it is the local supervising authority which has the power to suspend a midwife from practice in accordance with Council's rules and not the supervisor of midwives. Therefore no action will be taken by this Council on reports from supervisors of midwives.'

Every time a midwife is 'suspended' even if on further investigation that 'suspension' is declared void, it hurts our profession, it makes midwives feel intimidated, and our collective confidence is undermined.

To suspend a midwife is an extremely serious action - the sentences available to the Boards and Council are very limited and consist mainly of striking off or not striking off the register. No action should be undertaken lightly, especially as once the Board has been notified it cannot stop the proceedings against the midwife - they have to be seen through. It should never be used to 'teach someone a lesson' or in a conflict of clinical judgement.

Midwives universally need to support each other. At the International Confederation of Midwives I met supervisors of midwives who were trying to do that, who had stayed in the labour ward to support the midwife who was supporting a woman who was acting against medical advice, for example. Supervisors are part of the great sisterhood of midwifery, but when we have rules we must all follow them - none of us is above the law.

Reproduced with kind permission from Nursing Times, Vol. 83, No. 36 September 9, 1987

Supervision of Midwives

All midwives are allocated a supervisor to oversee their practice.
Independent midwife Caroline Flint presents her case against this system

Everyone in a professional role, whether lawyer, doctor, teacher or midwife, must be able to practice autonomously and use his or her professional judgement. However, with that freedom also comes a huge responsibility to the public and the necessity to earn the trust of those to whom the professional provides a service.

Within each service, therefore, a mechanism must exist whereby an aggrieved recipient of care or services can complain about the actions of the professional concerned and be assured that the professional will face some form of enquiry which may, if the fault is serious, lead to him or her being deprived of professional status.

For complaints against a solicitor, members of the public can contact the Law Society. The Royal Institute of British Architects is the body that deals with complaints against an architect. Complaints against a doctor are dealt with by the General Medical Council, and those against a midwife or nurse by the UKCC. All of this is right and proper, but for the midwives there is the potential for far greater scrutiny than this mechanism – via the supervision system.

One theory in favour of the supervision of midwives is that parents aggrieved at the care (or lack of care) they have received from their midwife have someone to complain to who is more accessible than a distant statutory body. In every health authority in the land there are, by statute, 'supervisors of midwives'. These august beings are there in a twofold role: to protect the public against unsafe midwifery practice but also to act as professional support to those midwives under their jurisdiction.

It sounds laudable, but it is an issue that causes passionate debate within the profession and not a few unfair situations. For instance, I believe, a woman can be happy with the care she has received from a midwife; the father can be happy with the care his partner has received; the baby can be healthy and well. The GP can be bowled over with admiration at the actions of the midwife. The hospital doctors can be happy to have worked with the midwife and respect what she has done. The midwife herself can feel she has done a good job. But at any time at all this same midwife may be summoned to see her supervisor and the care she has provided will be critically scrutinized by someone who was not there at the time and whose philosophy she may not share.

The system can, however, work to the midwife's advantage and leave her feeling extremely supported in her professional life. If the midwife has had a difficult experience – for instance, if a baby has been born extremely limp and unresponsive, very difficult to resuscitate – the midwife may be distressed and feel guilty, thinking it was her fault. The supervisor, eagle-eyed at detecting mistakes, goes through the documentation on the case and pronounces: 'As far as I can see there is no cause for criticism here. You acted appropriately at all times.' The midwife breathes again; her practice has been supported. She is not being blamed. But is this the best way of dealing with this type of problem?

With difficult obstetric and paedriatric cases the doctors present the case and the care they gave to a group of their peers and seniors. Mild admonishments follow. 'Well, if it had been me I would have done so-and-so. Did you consider doing...? Was there any evidence of...?'. The details are picked over by medical detectives at work, trying to piece together the full story, trying to learn how to do better next time. The midwife, on the other hand, is surveyed by a single supervisor and is therefore extremely vulnerable – whether or not further action is taken can depend on the supervisor seeing her point of view, on the supervisor being up to date clinically or on the supervisor remembering what it is like being at a home birth. This system can undermine midwives' confidence in their clinical ability. 'Supervision' should be regarded as a support mechanism enabling midwives to practice with confidence.

As a midwife specializing in home births I have often been relieved to talk over the phone to a supervisor who has soothed and supported me in difficult clinical situations. With a woman at home the midwife can feel isolated and afraid. The voice of a sympathetic supervisor over the phone can boost a midwife's confidence and lift her spirits. 'Could you negotiate with her to come into hospital if there has still been no progress in four hours' time?' Have you thought about a change of scenery and a piece of toast? That sometimes does the trick.' Another view can be all a midwife needs.

Supervisors of midwives have the right to inspect all equipment, all documentation, the premises from which the midwife practises and to scrutinize clients' notes. The principle is good, but the logistics can be ridiculous.

Our private practice is in central London. The M25 is our chosen boundary; consequently we register our 'Intention to Practise' in 28 different health authorities. In each health district there are four or five supervisors of midwives. We estimate that in our practice is supervised by at least 126 supervisors, all of whom have the right to inspect our equipment and scrutinize our registers and notes. We overcome this problem by inviting the supervisors to lunch every year – we hold two lunches over a two-week period because there are so many. The lunches are great fun, with them looking at our equipment, our records of study days attended, books read, our statistics and a presentation of how we work– but to have so many supervisors of midwives is a particular problem in independent practice.

Even more complications arise when we have booked a woman from one area who is going to have her baby in a hospital in another area. We need to negotiate with the supervisor in each area and, having done that, if the women then delivers at home we have further discussion and negotiation with the supervisor of the area in which the woman lives, having probably had much more discussion previously with the supervisor of the area in which the woman was going to deliver.

Midwives' practice is overseen by a book of rules. Questions arise over any profession which has a book containing a total of 44 rules, but the rule which is seen by many midwives as a catch-all is Rule 40. 'In any case where there is an emergency or where she detects in the health of a mother or baby a deviation from the norm a practising midwife shall call to her assistance a registered medical practitioner.'

This rule has come down almost unaltered from the 1902 Midwives Act when doctors did not want midwives to be autonomous practitioners, and the 1902 Act was only passed as long as doctors could be those people who ruled the profession and made up the majority of members of the Central Midwives' Board. This rule makes midwives vulnerable at every turn.

Obviously a thinking midwife will refer to a doctor in the case of an emergency that she cannot deal with herself or where there is an abnormality. But what is abnormal? Who defines abnormality?

If a woman is in labour at 37 weeks of pregnancy at home, is it normal or is it abnormal? If she is in labour at 36.5 weeks of pregnancy is it normal or is it abnormal? Who defines this. If she is a first-time mother and she is 35, is it normal or is it abnormal? If she is 44, is it normal or abnormal? Meconium staining occurs in about 25 per cent of women in labour. Is this normal or abnormal? If a baby is known to be presenting by the breech and the breech is emerging smoothly and well, is it a normal breech presentation or is it an abnormal delivery?

At the moment so many of our definitions of normality are based on obstetric criteria which may not always be relevant to the practice of midwifery.

The issues surrounding supervision need to be addressed by the profession. For this reason the Association of Radical Midwives has set up a working party to address them.

Reproduced with kind permission from Nursing Times, November 17, Volume 89, No 46 1993.

Why do Midwives want a New Act?

The Central Midwives Board

From 1902 until 1979 midwives in the United Kingdom had their own Statutory Body – for midwives in England and Wales it was the Central Midwives Board which was housed in the impressive Iolanthe House which had been the home of W.S Gilbert of the composing duet – Gilbert and Sullivan. The Scottish midwives had the Central Midwives Board for Scotland the Northern Ireland Council for Nurses and Midwives looked after midwifery in Northern Ireland.

The Central Midwives Board was made up of 14 members:

four appointed by the Minister of Health
four were doctors – one appointed by the Royal College of Physicians, one by the Royal College of Surgeons, one by the Royal College of Midwives and one by the Society of Apothecaries;
two were certified midwives appointed by the Royal College of Midwives;
four were appointed by (one each) the Queens Institute of District Nursing, the County Councils Association, the Association of Municipal Corporations and the Society of Medical Officers of Health.

Outnumbered midwives

For the whole of the Board's life midwives were always outnumbered, and it wasn't until 1965 that the Board was chaired by a midwife. The Central Midwives Board carried out several functions laid down in statute:

• The maintenance of a Roll of Certified Midwives.
• The removal from the Roll of Midwives who had been guilty of professional conduct.
• Approving courses of training for people wishing to become midwives.
• The disciplining of midwives who had a case of misconduct brought against them.
• Setting the standards for, and approving courses for Midwives' Refresher Courses.
• Setting standards of practice for midwives – which they did in two publications – the Midwives Rules and Guidance on the Midwives Code of Practice.

The Nurses, Midwives and Health Visitors Act 1979

In 1979, despite misgivings from several midwifery organizations the Central Midwives Board was replaced when the Nurses, Midwives and Health Visitors Act was passed and the National Boards for Nursing, Midwifery and Health Visiting were set up in the four countries of the United Kingdom. Heading this was the United Kingdom Central Council for Nursing, Midwifery and Health Visiting.

Doughty midwife campaigners had ensured the protection of the specific interests and needs of Midwifery by the inclusion of Statutory Midwifery Committees – both at Board and Council level. The Midwifery Committees were seen as the successors to the Central Midwives Board, the Council was responsible for maintaining the professional register and the eventual vision was to ensure that the register was an up to date register – which the midwives roll had always been, because of midwives' duty to register their intention to practise each year.

The Midwives' Roll had been the envy of the other professions because their Roll was the only one which was 'living'. The nurses roll contained everyone who had ever qualified as a nurse or health visitor and only those who had taken the trouble to inform the relevant body were removed at death or cessation of practice.

Standards of practice

The other duty of the Central Council was to establish standards of professional conduct for all the professions – as the Central Midwives Board had done since 1902 and to hold the Professional Conduct Committee which would be responsible for removing the names of miscreants from the Register. The Council was also to make statutory rules governing the entry to training and criteria for registration – their remit was also to improve the standards of training of all three professions.

The Central Council was to be made up of 45 members – of that number was to be one midwife from each National Board.

The four National Boards were to approve institutions which provided training/education courses for nurses, midwives and health visitors and control the examination system. The Boards also held the Investigating Committee to investigate charges of misconduct against a nurse, midwife or health visitor and refer to the Professional Conduct Committee at the United Kingdom Central Committee any serious cases.

The National Boards also held 45 members – five of those members were elected midwives. The midwives at both Board and Council level became members of the Midwifery Committees of either Board or Council, they were joined by some midwives who

were appointed by the Secretary of State and by the representatives of the medical, nursing and health visiting professions. For the first time ever, midwives formed the majority on their own governing body.

Doubts creep in

Despite the clause in the Nurses, Midwives and Health Visiting Act (7.3) 'Each Board shall consult its Midwifery Committee on all matters relating to midwifery and the Committee shall on behalf of the Board, discharge such of the Board's functions as are assigned to them by the Board or by the Secretary of State by order', the Midwifery Committee at Board level began to realize that even when they had agreed a matter which was in the interests of midwifery, the matter would be brought to the open Board and unless it was worded in such a way as to be acceptable to all the other members of the Board – could be outvoted.

The Act had not safeguarded the work of the Midwifery Committee at Board level in the way it had done to the Midwifery Committee at Council level in two clauses – 4.4 'The Secretary of State shall not approve rules relating to midwifery practice unless satisfied that they are framed in accordance with recommendations of the Council's Midwifery Council' and 4.5 'Any matter which is assigned to the Midwifery Committee otherwise than under Subsection 3 shall be finally dealt with by the Committee on behalf of the Council, so far as the Council expressly authorize the Committee to deal finally with it, and the Committee shall make a report to the Council as to the way in which they have dealt with the matter.'

Cracks in the system began to show up at the English National Board – despite the rule about 'consultation' with the Midwifery Committee, midwife members were becoming concerned that matters which they felt were relevant to their profession were being labelled 'management ' or 'administration' matters and by-passed the

Midwifery Committee. Also matters which were important to midwives were often discussed in 'closed' sessions of the Board and midwife members were warned that all matters discussed within the 'closed' session were highly confidential. It was whispered that to discuss such matters with any other person could constitute professional misconduct. During these closed sessions members of the press and visitors were excluded. The most important decisions about the midwifery profession were being taken in secret with Midwife members so intimidated that they dared not discuss them with the very people who had elected them.

A head-on clash came in 1989 when, against the expressed opposition of the Midwifery Committee, the Board decided that approval of midwifery, nursing and health visiting schools was to be performed by Education Officers who were 'generic' – i.e. that any education officer could approve any training school. That a Midwife Education Officer could approve a training school for nurses, or psychiatrically trained nurses and likewise an Education Officer who had a qualification in Mental Handicap nursing, or general nursing could approve a training school for midwives because all that they were 'approving' was the educational component.

At a stroke this destroyed the concept that in midwifery, education and practice are joined together – that midwifery is a practical skill and needs to be taught at the bedside as much as in the classroom. Midwifery Tutors had always expected to practise clinically in order to extend their students knowledge and skills, and likewise, all midwives saw themselves as teachers of those less experienced than themselves. It also lost midwives control over their own education.

Throughout Europe, midwifery and nursing have always been two separate and different professions – with their own individual training. In England, Direct Entry into midwifery has always been a way of entering the midwifery profession. The loss of control over their education increased when, despite very strong representation from midwives all over the country against being included in Project 2000 – which perceives midwifery as a specialist branch of nursing – most midwifery training schools are being incorporated into Colleges of Nursing – the name is being changed to 'College of Nursing and Midwifery' but as ever the midwives are outnumbered and their sphere of influence is dependent upon the loudness of the voice of the Senior Midwife Teacher.

Does it matter?

Is this just the bleating of a small profession which doesn't want to be overwhelmed by a larger, amorphous profession? It may just be that. On the other hand midwives are saying that if they disappear and become just another branch of nursing, women will be the ultimate losers. Midwives and nurses have fundamentally differing philosophies. Nurses are caring for the sick, and inevitably (except for a few practitioner nurses) that includes working with, and following the instructions of, doctors.

Midwives, on the other hand, are dealing with healthy women. They see part of their role as protecting women against the over enthusiastic ministrations of a medical profession who can find pathology around every corner – the rivalry between obstetricians and midwives is healthy and has a protective function for women. Midwives can take on a healthy woman who is pregnant and can provide full care for her throughout her pregnancy, labour and the puerperium. She can prescribe a limited range of drugs – such as pethidine, local anaesthetic, syntometrine and ergometrine, she can arrange ultrasound scans and blood tests. Unless the woman exhibits any deviations from normality, the midwife is not obliged to refer to a doctor at all – although most work in liaison with doctors.

The fact that few midwives take on the full range of midwifery practice is to be regretted, but that midwives should be seen, and see themselves as a separate and identifiable profession is probably to the benefit of women having babies. It has been noticed by several reporters that the Caesarean section rate rise in those countries where the midwifery profession is weak and see themselves as nurses because the over medicalization of childbirth carries on unabated with nurses acting out the doctors' wishes and no strong midwives to bring an atmosphere of reality into the labour ward.

A new Midwives Act

A group of midwives , together with mothers and members of the consumer groups have got together and with the help of a lawyer have drafted a new Bill for Midwives. This would set up a separate statutory body for midwives – called the Central Midwives Council and would ensure that midwives would be a strong and identifiable profession, that midwives would be judged in professional misconduct issues by midwives – not by nurses, and that midwives' education would be planned and approved by midwives.

The Royal College of Midwives has passed a motion to campaign for a new Midwives Act and has set up a Committee to look at ways of strengthening the midwifery profession within the present Act.

Many obstetricians regret the passing of the strong midwife – she may have been a rather bolshy individual, but she knew exactly what she was doing and she certainly saw her loyalty as lying with the women in her care. Midwives and Obstetricians have always worked together in a sometimes uneasy liaison, there are vested interests trying to destroy midwifery as a separate profession and midwives need the support of Obstetricians – it is they who can invariably see the strength of the midwives' argument.

Reproduced with kind permission from Obstetrics and Gynaecology Product News, Spring 1991

The Demise of the Midwifery Profession

What will happen to the midwifery profession if assessment and training become generic?

At last years' Annual General Meeting of the Royal College of Midwives, Margaret Brain, President of the Royal College of Midwives said in her speech to RCM members: 'As a profession we have the right to control and assess our own education and it is essential that we do so. In fact, if we lose control of our education we lose control of our profession.'

What did Margaret Brain know that the rest of us did not? What was causing her worries over midwives losing control over their education?

Generic education

Throughout last year rumours rumbled that the midwifery education officers at the English National Board (and at the other Boards) are now to be 'generic' and the Peat Marwick McLintock Report appears to take this aspect as having already happened.

What has happened for midwifery education officers is that they now can examine and approve mental handicap training schools or health visiting establishments.

What about midwifery education establishments? They are about to be visited and assessed by nurses who have never qualified let alone practised as midwives. Midwives' education will be assessed by nurses who are no doubt superb at assessment and evaluating district nursing, maybe psychiatric nursing or general nursing, but who will probably have no perception that the pregnant woman is a healthy individual who has no need to be in hospital and who has rights and needs which are totally different from all other members of a hospital's population who are always there because there is something 'wrong 'with them. It is all very well to separate the education of nurses, midwives and health visitors and lump it under the name 'education' and there may be good arguments in strengthening the educational input of professional officers, but to expect midwifery training schools to be assessed by people other than midwives means that indeed midwives have lost control of their profession. The next step is that midwifery itself will disappear and midwives will become post graduate nurses or obstetric nurses.

Home and abroad

The precedent for this is all around us. It has happened in New Zealand, Australia, Japan, India, Scotland – in many states of America midwives are illegal, and in Canada midwives have just been having a tremendous fight to become legalized. Here in the United Kingdom we have had a wonderful legal framework for midwifery ever since 1902. Midwives felt that they were protected by the paragraph in the 'Nurses, Midwives and Health Visitors Act' 1979 which states: 'Each board shall consult its Midwifery Committee on all matters relating to midwifery and the Committee shall, on behalf of the Board, discharge such of the Board's functions as are assigned to them by the Board or by the Secretary of State by order' (7(3)). In law this means that the Board cannot disregard the consultation with the Midwifery Committee, but, as Board Midwife Mary Cronk pointed out at the Board Meeting on Tuesday 14th November, despite consultation the Board can totally ignore and ride roughshod over the expressed wishes of the Midwifery Committee.

The Midwifery Committee fought hard battles to prevent the 'generalization' of the midwifery education officers. This is the same Midwifery Committee which only two years ago stated that midwifery education must ensure that midwifery remains 'a separately identifiable profession'.

What about the paragraph in the Nurses, Midwives and Health Visitors Act (1979) which states 'The Secretary of State shall not approve rules relating to midwifery practice unless satisfied that they are framed in accordance with recommendations of the Council's Midwifery Committee' (4(4))? Is the Midwifery Committee of the UKCC happy about this action? I can hardly believe it.

Apprenticeship training

Midwifery education has always been different from even the most basic principles of nursing education, and now that nursing education is becoming more and more college-based this divide is increasing. Midwife teachers have always had a high clinical input and links between service and education in midwifery have always been extremely close. Midwifery is almost an 'apprentice' training, with the student midwife learning practically with an experienced midwife or midwife teacher. The reason that we have never seen a need for 'Clinical Teachers' in midwifery is because we have always argued that all midwives are 'Clinical Teachers' including midwife teachers.

It is notable that in most midwifery units the midwifery education department is within the service area. Although this often means that the Midwifery Education Department is cramped and stuck in a small space, it does ensure that the education of midwives happens in a practical setting, that theory is always based on practice and that midwifery teachers are always available to the service midwives and indeed frequently provide a welcome ear for disgruntled or worried midwives to act as a guide and supporter when difficult clinical problems are tackled.

Until now, experienced midwives have assessed midwifery training schools. They have been acutely aware of the clinical input that the students receive and the English National Board approval of training has been held up while a deficit in clinical practice has been rectified. This has given great help to the clinicians and managers who have been able to improve service despite financial cutbacks. Without this impetus the training school would not have been approved.

Legal implications

It is now time for the midwifery profession to look at the legal implications of this action by the English National Board. If the midwifery profession is being deprived of midwives assessing and approving its training then a profession is being destroyed. There has to be recourse to the law by way of judicial review. It is not in the interests of the women of the United Kingdom that the midwifery profession should disappear. It is up to the midwifery professional bodies to act on behalf of the profession to ensure that midwifery education is assessed by midwives.

Reproduced with kind permission from Midwife, Health Visitor and Community Nurse, March 1990, Vol. 26, No. 3

Requiem for Midwifery

No more midwifery education officers
In a letter dated 11th October 1989 Anthony Smith, 'Director - Education Policy Implementation' of the English National Board for Nursing, Midwifery and Health Visiting has written to all senior midwifery tutors to inform them that in future there will be a 'development' in the role of education officers. Each education officer will work with a number of institutions across the entire range of courses for the training of nurses, midwives and health visitors - this 'development' to come into operation on 1st April 1990.

The implications of this 'development' are that midwifery training schools will from April 1990 be assessed for approval or re-approval by 'generic' educational officers. Thus a midwifery training school may be assessed by a general trained nurse education officer, or a health visitor trained education officer, or a mental handicap nurse trained education officer. Probably no one could fault any of these education officers in their education component, and this might be acceptable if midwifery education was all about education. If the education officers were only approving the educational component of midwifery training having generic education officers might be acceptable, but midwifery training and education has always been service based and herein lies its greatest strength. Student midwives learn most of what they do by example. They learn some of their knowledge in the classroom but a large part of classroom teaching is consolidation of that which has been learnt in the ward or community.

Midwives have always (except in Scotland) resisted the notion of 'clinical teachers' because most midwife tutors see their role as teaching by example in the clinical situation.

The effects of having 'generic' education officers assessing midwifery training schools could have a catastrophic effect on the way women are cared for. Despite assurances that the 'generic' education officers will have access to 'specialist advice' from education officers who are trained midwives, they will not be going round maternity units with the eye of a midwife. We have said until our throats are dry that midwifery is different from nursing, that when a nurse looks after a patient that patient has to have by very definition 'something wrong' with them. In midwifery it is not like that – women we care for have nothing 'wrong' with them, they are healthy individuals who need support and empowering, not to be 'cared for' even in the kindest fashion.

Ever since the Central Midwives' Board was set up at the beginning of the century we have had midwifery education officers who are trained and previously practising midwives. They have seen what the undercurrents are in a midwifery training school. Many a school has been buoyed up by the words from the education officer 'I shall not recommend this school for re-approval unless...'. The unless has varied according to each school, it may be that the school will not be recommended unless they get more secretarial help, or books for the library, but it can also be that the recommendations will be withheld until the obstetricians stop being so interventionist in their management of labouring women and allow the midwives to practise as midwives , or it may be that the labour ward is so unpleasant for women to have a baby in that the school will not be recommended for re-approval until the place has become more appropriate for the accommodation of labouring women, or that untrained personnel are no longer allowed to give advice on breast feeding, or that obstetricians must stop seeing all pregnant women themselves and must allow some of the women to be seen by the midwives.

The effect of education officers with both practical and theoretical midwifery skills has meant a definite improvement in the climate for pregnant women, the gains in both 'humanizing' of labour wards and antenatal clinics has been great, and the awareness of the midwife of her skills and role has been increased by the midwifery education officers

Midwifery committee overruled

The other frightening aspect of this edict from the English National Board is that it has been sprung on us unawares (obviously deliberate). Where has the debate been? Where has the consultation either with the bodies representing midwives, or with the profession? For an elected body to deliberately cut off its electorate , to withhold information from those who voted for them is appalling. The midwife members of the Board have been looking preoccupied for several months; when asked what is the matter they have only replied 'I can't tell you, it's confidential'. The English National Board took the decision to do away with midwifery education officers and replace them with generic education officers against the expressly stated opposition of the midwifery committee. This has forced the Chairman of the midwifery

committee to take the unprecedented step of issuing a public statement to publicize the opposition of the midwifery committee to this measure. 'The committee do not believe this policy change to be beneficial to the midwifery profession'.

The midwifery committee chairman's statement goes on 'The English National Board's Midwifery Committee clearly and unequivocally opposed the concept of Education Officers undertaking a generic role, on the basis that it was a radical movement away from a proven specialist support mechanism for integrated midwifery education and practice'. The midwives we elected to the midwifery committee have been ignored , the discussions have taken place behind closed doors. One wonders how or why our elected members have been so intimidated that they have not been able to share their concerns and anxieties with their electorate.

But most worrying of all is that a principle fundamental to midwifery education has been steamrollered by the very body which has the remit to improve midwifery education. When the UKCC was founded in 1979 midwives expressed their concern that midwives' interests would be lost to the numerically superior nurses. To ally these fears, provision was made in the 1979 Nurses, Midwives and Health Visitors Act 'that each board shall consult its midwifery committee on all matters relating to midwifery'. We now have a concrete example of this consultation process being woefully inadequate to safeguard the midwifery profession when the nursing majority holds a different view.

Perhaps it is time to take up the cry 'MIDWIVES OUT OF THE STATUTORY BODIES' because we are certainly being destroyed by them.

An original article commissioned by MIDIRS, December 1989.

The Golden Thread

In 1935 the then Lord Chancellor, Viscount Sankey, delivered a judgement and coined a phrase which has become famous - 'Throughout the web of the English Criminal Law one golden thread is always to be seen, that it is the duty of the prosecution to prove the prisoner's guilt.' In fact this principle has always been so strongly observed in English Law that until the beginning of this century the accused was not allowed to give evidence himself - in case he damned himself from his own lips - it was always the job of the prosecution to prove his guilt, not the accused job to prove his innocence.

There are two other 'golden threads' which make up the Common Law of England and the concept of 'natural justice' and those are that the accused has a right to know what s/he is charged with - and that s/he should have a right to be heard, a right to clear his/her name by giving his/her side of the story.

I am becoming increasingly concerned about these principles of justice as they apply to midwives.

In our Professional Conduct Machinery there is room for all these principles to be upheld - but in practice these principles are being ignored to the detriment of several midwives - who like any other member of the English public is entitled to justice.

To start at the beginning - any member of the public or profession may report a midwife for alleged professional misconduct to the Investigating Committee of the English National Board, but in practice the whole process is usually initiated by the midwife's Supervisor of Midwives.

To digress for a second - the role of the Supervisor of Midwives is a facet of our profession which we really need to be addressing. The Supervisor of Midwives is seen as 'Guide, Counsellor and Friend' to the midwives over whom she has supervision. When she is actually acting as guide, counsellor and friend her role is supportive and that of the 'wise and experienced' mentor to the midwives in her care. She is also there to ensure that the public are being offered care of a satisfactory and safe standard. She is not there as the relentless critic of every midwife under her control.

All other professionals have two professional relationships - their relationship with their client and their relationship with their professional body. We midwives also have these professional relationships - but in addition we have a third person who can intervene in this relationship - the Supervisor of Midwives. Many midwives see the supervisor as the 'safeguard' of our profession and there is no doubt that having the role of supervisor enacted in statute has helped the profession against some of the greater excesses of the Griffiths reforms - but what about our profession? Is the role of supervisor really helpful to us professionally? Is this extra tier in our professional relationship a support or a heavy weight dragging us back from being truly professional? Infantilizing us? Are we the only professionals who need a 'nanny' to make sure that we don't harm Josephine Public? And what about Josephine Public? Is she really being protected from incompetent midwifery by the Supervisor of Midwives? In some cases the answer must be 'yes', but is this only because we have supervisors when any member of the public can report a midwife? Are all midwives who are not professionally up to scratch in front of the Professional Conduct Committee? The answer has to be 'No', and in fact it could be seen that in practice the reverse happens - that the midwives who speak out and who are less able to be 'controlled' because they practise outside the normal system appear to be under much greater threat of being involved in professional disciplinary actions than their more submissive counterparts.

The other worrying factor of the professional disciplinary machinery of nurses, midwives and health visitors is that the practitioner can have an unblemished professional record, can have been an excellent clinician all her working life and as the result of one inadvertent slip can be struck off the register. The injustice of this was pointed out by Lord Justice Watkins VC recently when a school nurse, Elizabeth Hefferon appealed to the High Court against the decision to strike her off the register by the UKCC Professional Conduct Committee after one inadvertent slip - freely admitted at the time. The High Court quashed her striking-off and highly criticised the procedures of the Professional Conduct Committee.

To return to my initial hypothesis - that natural justice may be being denied to midwives -

A midwife may be suspended from practice by her Local Supervising Authority on the advice of the Supervisor - can deprive her of her professional identity, deprive her of her livelihood - *without ever having spoken to the midwife concerned, without ever having corresponded with the midwife concerned and without ever having given her an opportunity to give her side of the story.*

If the midwife is suspended from practice the case against her must be reported to the Investigating Committee of the English National Board, she will receive a letter from the Investigations Department as will any midwife who has been reported to the English National Board - 'Information has been received at the Board containing allegation(s) of misconduct against yourself', but what are the allegation(s)? Is it one or twenty? Is it a case the midwife conducted three weeks ago or a woman she delivered ten years ago? What are the charges she is being asked to answer?

Here is the other aspect of the procedure which I suggest contravenes all concepts of natural justice - it can be WEEKS before she knows the charges against her, the sword of Damocles hangs over her head, daily she awaits its drop.

Another aspect which causes concern is the conduct of the Investigating Committee - the case against the midwife (who by now had an opportunity to hear the case against her and to give a written reply) is perused by the Investigating Committee - *who feel quite at liberty to add extra charges – despite the fact that the midwife is not present, nor is her representative, to answer the additional charges.*

All the charges can now be taken to the Professional Conduct Committee which is conducted like a court "Save as aforesaid and where provided in these rules all proceedings before the Conduct Committee shall take place in the presence of all parties thereto who appear therein and *shall be open to the public...*" (16(2) - this is all very well but have you ever tried to gain access to a Professional Conduct Hearing? You have to write and apply for tickets before being allowed access. Are the tickets given out fairly? Are certain names not sent tickets? If access is only by ticket, can it really be said that the hearing is open to the public?

Professional Conduct Machinery is the responsibility of the profession - how responsible are we being with ours?

Reference
1. The Nurses, Midwives and Health Visitors (Professional Conduct) Rules 1987, Approval Order 1987, Statutory Instrument No. 2156 from HMSO.

Reproduced with kind permission from The Association of Radical Midwives Magazine, Summer, 1988 Issue No. 37.

Rules for Midwives

The UKCC is in the process of formulating a set of regulations that will govern the future practice of midwifery in this country. Caroline Flint suggests that the new rules will influence the pattern of childbearing for years to come

The UKCC is asking the midwives of Great Britain to help them to formulate rules which will last us (and the mothers and babies of our lands) well into the next century. What the midwives decide *now* will affect child bearing for decades to come. It is essential that we get it right.

Midwives are meeting throughout the country to discuss the proposed rules sent out for consultation. What will they decide? How can they get it right?

For many midwives, the words in the code of practice attached to the Central Midwives Board handbook, issued following the Midwives Act 1951, have been a constant inspiration : 'The Midwives Act 1951 gives statutory recognition to the position of the midwife as a professional practitioner in her own right.'

Most midwives in 1984 are very deeply committed to the ideal of the midwife as a 'professional practitioner' able to practise using her full skills for the benefit and support of the women, babies and families in her care.

But one problem is that the skills of the midwife are frequently intangible while the skills of the obstetrician are tangible.

So what do midwives need in their rules to enable them to practise as 'professional practitioners'? What do women need defined in the midwives' rules to enable them to have a safe experience of childbirth? What do obstetricians need defined in our rules so that they can leave us to get on with the provinces that are ours?

The *Principles for formulation of the new rules* as formulated in the consultation paper are refreshing and forward looking:

1. There should be a fresh approach to the formulation of new rules.

2. The wording of the rules should be clear, concise and comprehensible.

3. In order to allow practical application throughout the United Kingdom the rules should be as broad as is consistent with legal requirements.

4. The rules should define the level of professional responsibility of the midwife.

5. While safeguarding standards of care the rules should permit professional development and not inhibit changes which would be desirable as knowledge increases and practice and attitudes change.

With these inspiring words ringing in my ears I am struck with delight when I read in the section on spheres of practice and levels of responsibility that the midwifery committee considers that a midwife should be required, at all times, to give care to women and babies on her own responsibility when there are no complications, and she should give this care in co-operation with registered medical practitioners where there are complications present. So far so good, but now my heart gives a little dive as the next two words are 'or anticipated'.

The beginning of this proposed rule is exciting and enables me to practise fully as a midwife. The middle of it is necessary and reasonable, but what about complications which are *anticipated*.

Does not this lead us back down the slippery slope to the very destructive philosophy 'that childbirth is only normal in retrospect'. This was mentioned in *The Role of the Midwife* by the now extinct central midwives boards, as the main threat to the execution of the role of the midwife.

Some people could *anticipate* complications in 95 per cent of the women we care for. I cannot feel that these words will be helpful either to midwives or to women.

The other specific section that worries me is section 5.9, 'The duty of the midwife when engaged to attend a home confinement'. As a profession we need to acknowledge that it is the small group of determined women who have carried on insisting on having their babies at home, who have saved midwifery from extinction. So I am sad to read in the proposed rules that, 'In view of the difficulties which may occur for midwives when engaged to attend a home confinement and the increasing demand by women for this service, the midwifery committee considered that there could be merit in having a rule on this subject. Such a rule would require a midwife to:

1. Carry out the policy of the local supervising authorities (LSAs).

2. Inform the woman's registered medical practitioner and the supervisor of midwives if she deems that home confinement is unsuitable.

3. Continue the care of the woman and her baby(ies), *unless otherwise instructed by the supervisor of midwives.'*

What happens to the midwife if the woman she is caring for wants something that is contravened in the LSA policy? Her first duty as a professional is to her client, but what if she incurs disciplinary action by putting her client's interests first? LSA policies vary from authority to authority. This suggestion could put the midwife in a very delicate position.

A midwife as a professional has obligations. That obligation includes providing care to a woman who requests care at home, in the same way a lawyer is obliged to defend someone who is on trial even though he or she may not wish to, or may think that the defendant is guilty. A professional person has obligations which cannot be removed by anyone, including the supervisor of midwives.

Reproduced with kind permission from Nursing Times, August 15, 1984

A Mother's Birthright

A government-backed report on maternity services has been given a mixed reception by midwives. Caroline Flint, midwifery sister at St George's Hospital, Tooting, looks at the report in detail

'A mother is not necessarily a "patient" and should not be referred to as such.' With the philosophy that underlies these words the Maternity Services Advisory Committee is leading midwives, obstetricians and the GPs of this country into the next decade of partnership with the childbearing population of women and their partners.

Its refreshing 'guide to good practice and plan for action', makes the woman having her baby in hospital the pivot, the axis around whom we should base our care. The care suggested is refreshingly sane and humane, avoiding the excesses produced by the philosophy that 'childbirth is only safe in retrospect'. It treads a flexible road which can bend to encompass the needs of the 'healthy woman for whom labour and birth are important physiological and emotional events,' as well as catering for those who need emergency and medical care.

While the sections relating to birth in hospital can be welcomed, sadly the one on birth at home is weak and dictatorial. However, let us dwell first on the excellent points of this document and look at how a woman can expect to be cared for in a hospital which implements all the suggestions in the report.

Tour of labour ward

During her pregnancy, the woman 'should have been given the opportunity to familiarize herself with the unit's environment - and to have met the staff who are likely to care for her'. If the woman finds it difficult to come during normal working hours, the report recommends that arrangements should be made to enable her to come and see the unit and 'discuss care during labour with the staff' at a time convenient to her.

Birth plan

The report recommends a 'birth plan' with the words, 'every mother should have the opportunity to discuss and agree an individual plan for her care during labour and childbirth'.

The suggested topics a woman might like to discuss in relation to her birth plan are: the role the father is to play during labour and delivery, pain relief, fetal monitoring, the position the mother wishes to adopt during labour and delivery, the mother's first contact with the baby, procedures if complications arise and feeding the baby.

Discussion

The birth plan and any worries during pregnancy are to be discussed when the woman comes to an antenatal appointment and 'she should be given opportunities for private discussion during clinics'.

Having had the opportunity to discuss in private how she would like her labour conducted, and these preferences having been written in her case notes, what will greet the labouring woman coming into hospital?

Welcome and continuity

When the woman arrives at the labour ward, someone will be there to welcome her. She will be then be allocated a midwife who will stay with her until the end of her shift. The midwife will not give her an enema or pubic shave unless she requests it (or unless it is medically advisable). I question the necessity of putting this recommendation in the report, four years after midwife Mona Romney's research findings were published on enemas and shaves, though, as I am sure no reasonable maternity units have been shaving women or giving them enemas during the past few years.

Privacy

In the chapters dealing with labour the report lays further emphasis on privacy. 'No-one should enter her room unnecessarily', and if the unit is a teaching unit 'the mother's agreement should be obtained before any students are allowed into her room'. Her husband should not be asked to leave the room during examinations if he and the mother are content for him to stay.

Midwives

Midwives will be relieved to hear that 'decisions about the care of individual mothers should be taken by the midwife immediately responsible'. The senior midwife in overall charge should have a broad picture of all mothers in labour but the responsibility for care lies with the midwife staying with the mother. The midwife's role is very traditional - 'with woman' - and very supportive. Here are some examples:
• 'Mothers who do not wish to have any analgesics should be supported in this aim
• 'Episiotomy should not be performed routinely or without the mother's consent.'
• 'Some mothers dislike the idea of electronic monitoring, especially if it restricts their mobility or involves the artificial rupture of the membranes and the attachment of an electrode to the baby's scalp. If the mother does not accept the form of monitoring recommended, this should be recorded in her notes and her wishes respected.'
• 'During delivery, the mother should adopt the position which she feels is the most comfortable and effective.'

• 'Normally the midwife will be the key person supporting the mother. At the end of her shift she should hand over care to another midwife in the mother's presence.'

Doctors

The report suggests that 'there should be a doctor immediately available for the delivery suite'. In theory, this is a welcome suggestion, but in practice what does the bored doctor do while he hangs around the delivery suite waiting for an emergency to brew? Perhaps he is going through the birth register collecting statistics of obstetric procedures and their outcomes! This welcome suggestion comes in order 'to assist clinicians in the assessment of their practice', to be collected by the regional health authority and issued to the districts.

Drugs

The tone of the report becomes dogmatic when dealing with oxytocic drugs. 'The use of oxytocic drugs to aid early expulsion of the placenta and reduce the loss of blood after birth is normal practice. It is beneficial and mothers should be encouraged to accept it.' The pros and cons of using oxytocic drugs is outlined by Midwife Sally Inch in her book *Birthrights.*[1]

Operational policies

More dogma sadly creeps in here, ostensibly to 'ensure a consistent standard of care and avoid any confusion over practice' but it is, as ever, 'midwifery by numbers'. Guidelines are acceptable but policies written in minute detail are for unthinking automatons, not for practitioners who are trying to give individual care to a unique woman experiencing a unique labour. The danger of these kinds of policies is that they tend to make us behave like unthinking automatons, which it is quite clear this report doesn't really want.

There is also a chapter on design of the delivery suite - the usual suggestions of wallpaper and curtains are included, and 'adjustable beds'. Since the whole philosophy behind this report is to make birth as pleasant and as 'homelike' as possible, surely the labour ward would look much more 'homelike' with an ordinary double bed in it? (It would also be cheaper than any adjustable bed.) A conventional delivery bed can always be wheeled in if necessary.

Home births

Sadly this report refers to women who wish to have their babies at home almost as deviants. 'Some mothers might prefer to have their babies at home, despite the possible risks,' it says. Did anyone outline the risks of hospital births to those women having their babies in hospital? Doctors and midwives, placed in the role of policemen, might sometimes 'feel it their duty to try and persuade the mother to change her mind but they must recognise that the final decision is hers.' Happily the committee realises that 'health authorities have an obligation to see that a midwifery service is available for home births and that every district should have midwives available to attend home births who undertake a sufficient number of deliveries each year to maintain their confidence and skills.'

Some women choose home births because they are responsible and so concerned about their baby's entry into the world that they dare not risk letting their precious child be delivered and looked after by strangers. Increasingly it is becoming evident that for low risk women, birth at home is a valid choice, and in the current economic climate, two days in hospital (at least £200) can only compare unfavourably with the most expensive community midwife in your home for 24 hours (£40).

I'm sad that no mention has been made in the report of the desirability of having a midwife with a woman in labour who she has been able to get to know during her pregnancy. I am also sad that no mention was made of the huge difference it makes to women to be able to wear their own clothes during labour and to have their own pillows on the labour ward bed. However, the main theme of this report is useful, sensible and sensitive.

Reference
1. Inch, S. (1982). *Birthrights*. London: Hutchinson.

Reproduced with kind permission from Nursing Times, February 22, 1984

Getting it Right for Mother and Baby

Caroline Flint, SRN, SCM, Community Midwife examines some of the recommendations made by the Social Services Committee to improve the baby mortality rate

'A charter for mothers and babies in the coming years' is how the Social Services Committee, chaired by Renée Short, sees its list of 152 recommendations, on perinatal and neonatal mortality.

Its report points out that the mortality of infants in the first four years of life is twice as high in women who attend late for antenatal care, and that women who default from antenatal clinics after initially booking often have high-risk pregnancies. One of the first recommendations is that 'every effort should be made to encourage women to attend as early as possible in their pregnancies for antenatal care. In future the responsibility for bringing mothers with high-risk pregnancies to local clinics or general practitioner obstetricians for antenatal care should lie more with health visitors, community midwives and social workers than at present.'

The committee believes that the best incentive to bring mothers to the antenatal clinic or to their GP early in pregnancy is to make them aware of the advantages of antenatal care to themselves and particularly to their babies.

The report discusses the practical problems that many high-risk women have in getting to antenatal clinics - such as other children to look after or a long distance to travel, or social problems or fears of hospitals and clinical procedures - and when they finally arrive at the antenatal clinic, the picture the report paints is bleak '...cattle truck atmosphere, little privacy, little dignity, long waiting times, lack of continuity of care, lack of opportunity to discuss things that women themselves are worried about and the feeling that they are going through a rather mechanistic process and not getting out of it as much as they feel they should.'

The Committee recognizes that many hospital doctors and midwives are worried about the conditions in their clinics and that there is a very real need 'for guidelines for medical staffing, the number of midwives, nurses and clerical officers required for adequate staffing of an antenatal clinic.' It suggests that more use should be made of experienced midwives whose skills at present tend to be under-used. Often the midwife tends to prepare the patient for the doctor - i.e. by taking her blood pressure and weighing her - but leaves abdominal palpitation to the doctor, and this increases the wait the patient has at the clinic and also splits up the continuity of care the woman experiences in that clinic.

The report underlines time and again the importance of the midwife: 'It is impossible to overestimate the value to the maternity services of a group of individuals such as midwives who are dedicated to the care of mother and baby. We also recognize the greater cost-effectiveness of having midwives rather than obstetricians looking after normal, pregnant women who comprise the major part of the maternity population.

'We strongly recommend that every effort is made to re-establish midwifery as a profession that offers attractive prospects. We also recommend that a national recruiting campaign should be initiated to encourage newly qualified nurses to train in midwifery. This should also be directed at midwives who have left the service but are able to come back into practice. For the latter group it will be necessary to ensure that a sufficient number of suitable posts are available for married women who have a family to look after. Consideration should also be given to increasing 'direct' entry into midwifery as occurs in many countries in Europe.'

These words will be good news for the many women who are fired with enthusiasm for a career in midwifery by the miracle of their own birthing experiences and who have so far been deterred by the fact that at present they have to train as a nurse before they can begin their midwifery training (except for a very few schools in the country). It will also be good news for those mothers who already have their midwifery qualification and who have had difficulty in finding a post which fits in with their family commitments - many hospitals run most imaginative schemes for using the skills of the part-timer and perhaps such schemes will become more widespread following this report.

Many midwives believe that a much greater degree of continuity of care could be achieved within the present system, but it takes a degree of vision, openness and forward planning which may be difficult to achieve when most midwives feel snowed under with work because they are working in units which are, for the most part, short of staff. As one of the witnesses to the Committee said: 'Most of us do work longer hours, longer than the 40 hours we are supposed to work.' Another said: 'Staff become very unhappy at work due to poor staffing levels consequently (leading) to more staff leaving...'

Part of the report that troubled me greatly was the list of witnesses who gave evidence to the Committee. We are here concerned with a totally female function. The attendants on a woman during 75 per cent of births in this country are female, yet over twice as many men gave evidence to the Committee as did women. We need to realise that childbirth is a totally female activity, and

that it may be counter-productive to have men who are strangers involved in this activity.

Of course the vast majority of women want, and need, the man they love to be with them throughout the antenatal period, during labour and delivery and during the puerperium. But the involvement of men during childbirth needs to be looked at much more deeply than we have looked at it before and the opinions of men concerning childbirth can only be secondhand.

Thus, one of the recommendations in the report fills me with some foreboding: 'We recommend that there should be a 50 per cent expansion of the consultant grade in obstetrics and gynaecology over the next five years.'

Each consultant has a registrar and at least one house officer. Of course, some of them may be women, but how many? Does this not presage yet more male involvement and perhaps interference?

The report is very exciting in many ways in that it seems to have given official recognition to the emotional needs of parturient and postnatal women which may well be as important to the outcome of labour as their physical needs.

The use of drugs in labour was apparently out of the sphere of this report, except for 'We recommend that a 24-hour service for epidural anaesthesia should be available as an important priority in consultant obstetric units. In units where anaesthetists are unable to provide a 24-hour service, consideration should be given by anaesthetists to training obstetricians in the technique.'

The report points out that probably the lives of about 5,000 babies a year could be saved and that many deaths are caused by birth asphyxia. We know that all drugs appear to have some effect on the baby. We are using Phenergan and Sparine in a vast number of labours and we apparently have very little knowledge of their effects on the newborn; we use a great deal of pethidine which we know is a respiratory depressant, we also use a large number of epidurals.

Whether the local anaesthetic used has a direct effect on the neonate is, at the moment, uncertain. But the use of epidurals has direct implication on the outcome of many labours. Perhaps we should be looking at why women in this country need so much analgesia with all its implications for their babies, and whether by doing something different we might reduce the need for analgesia.

The newest data from the Office of Population Censuses and Surveys on perinatal mortality by place of birth is quoted by the report, showing an increase in perinatal mortality in home deliveries between 1976 and 1977, and the Committee recommends 'that home delivery be phased out further'.

Here, I think, the Committee needs to look further at the figures in question. When women want to have a baby at home they have to seek out a midwife and GP willing to take them on. Since 1970 and the Peel Report this has become almost impossible in many areas, so now if a woman wants a home confinement she often has a hard task on her hands.

If she is articulate and strong in her resolve she will seek out a midwife and GP often with the help of her local National Childbirth Trust Branch, or Society to Support Home Confinements. She may well have a hard task ahead of her and end up accepting a domino delivery or a home confinement perhaps grudgingly taken on, with her having to sign various forms to say that she takes on full responsibility for the outcome of her confinement, etc.

If she is not so strong, nor so articulate, nor so well informed, she may well just opt out all together and stay at home receiving no antenatal care and dialling 999 when the birth of her baby is imminent. The figures for both the former and the latter are all lumped together as 'home confinements', and my premise is that the latter group is growing rapidly and will grow if we make no humane provision for them.

Home delivery should not be phased out any further. It is almost non-existent now in many areas, and however much we 'humanize' hospitals, however welcoming and loving the staff, however often we suggest that women should give birth in consultant units, however much we appeal to reason and statistics, there will always be women who really cannot give birth in hospital.

I also suggest we are placing many women at risk because we are denying them the medical care they need when they quite categorically refuse hospital delivery. It must always be safer to book a home delivery and have all necessary equipment available and the hospital and flying squad alerted, than to be called out in the middle of the night to an unbooked woman who has had no antenatal care, no available history, no phone in the house, whose baby can be presenting in an abnormal way and who can be anaemic.

We often say that women get too emotional when talking about birth - the campaigners for home confinement often are accused of this - but we are talking about a subject which must be an emotional issue for women.

But it is no wonder women become emotional about the place of birth; the whole of parturition is so intrinsically bound up in a woman's emotional and sexual feelings that figures will always tend to be somewhat irrelevant to women.

'A charter for mothers and babies' - yes, up to a point. A charter for obstetricians - yes. A charter for anaesthetists - definitely. A charter for midwives - yes. Let's hope it makes us all think and act on our thoughts, because only then will it really become 'A charter for mothers and babies in the coming years'.

Reproduced with kind permission from Nursing Mirror, August 7 1980

There but for the Grace of God go I

We often say it when we hear about someone going before the Professional Conduct Committee or sometimes we only think it very quietly so that no one else will know 'There but for the grace of God go I'. But is this what we really should be thinking? When I walk past the Old Bailey, or even for that matter when I walk past my local Coroners Court do I think 'There but for the grace of God go I'? Do we say to ourselves 'Thank goodness I haven't mugged any old ladies recently', or 'I'm relieved that I have restrained myself from committing any frauds in the last few months', or 'Thank goodness I've managed to avoid murdering anyone this year'? Of course not, we don't have to restrain ourselves from mugging old ladies or from committing violent crimes because they are something that is totally outside our normal behaviour - we don't say 'There but for the grace of God go I' because the sort of behaviour that comes before the courts is totally outside normal behaviour and is outside our sphere of experience. Actions which come before a court of law, a Criminal Court, are not those we would contemplate in our everyday lives.

But does the same principle hold for our professional Conduct Committee? Should it be possible for me to think when I hear about the behaviour of a fellow nurse, midwife or health visitor who is facing censure and trial from the Professional Conduct Committee 'There but for the grace of God go I'? Because if it is possible for me to say that to myself, it must surely mean that the mores of the Committee are too severe? If I can see

exactly how a certain professional was able to do what he/she did, indeed I could have been there myself, surely we are not talking about totally unreasonable behaviour? Are we not talking about the sort of behaviour that any reasonable professional might exhibit under the stresses experienced by the professional at that time?

Is it right for our professional conduct machinery to be trying those professionals who are acting in a way that is not totally unreasonable? Surely this means that if any one of us makes an error in clinical judgement, or if any one of us makes an inadvertent slip, or if any one of us makes a genuine mistake we could be up before the Professional Conduct Committee and fighting or our professional lives? It is right and just that the professional conduct machinery should protect the public because nurses, midwives and health visitors have a duty to their clients to give safe and professional care, but if they never ever make a mistake surely the standard set is perhaps too high?

The reasoning behind the philosophy that no-one should ever make a mistake also gives too much power to the managers of that particular health professional - 'Now Nurse Roberts, you've given the wrong drug to Baby Jones - I won't report you THIS time but from now on I want to hear no more complaints about how my ward is run. You don't have a leg to stand on any more.' A farfetched suggestion? Probably, but I'm sure you can fill in the scenario yourself, if every health professional is afraid of making even the tiniest mistake, and even more if every health professional is afraid of having even the tiniest mistake discovered - this encourages dishonesty, a reluctance to admit to a misdemeanour, subterfuge, surely not healthy in a profession which is trying to be more and more accountable?

The other thought I would like you to explore is which professionals usually come before the Professional Conduct Committee - it is not the manager, nor is it the educationalist - it is invariably the clinician. Now this may seem obvious because it is the actions of clinicians which have the most immediate effect on the population at large but does this mean that to ensure that I don't come before the Professional Conduct Committee, it is essential that I leave clinical practice? Is it right? Should I be more vulnerable as a clinician? Or is my vulnerability inevitable? It does seem rather hard that as a clinician I not only receive less salary than a manager or educationalist, but also I am more likely to be involved in professional conduct machinery which is always stressful, always painful, always time-consuming, and which leaves the professional involved with a stigma for ever - even if she is vindicated. Actually she is never vindicated, she is 'Let off' - she is referred to the rules, or the judgement on her case is postponed, or she is told that there is no case to answer. Notwithstanding the effects are felt by her professionally for the rest of her career. 'There's the midwife who was up before the UKCC two years ago' is whispered as she walks by. Mud sticks and even if she has had an exemplary career and on one occasion only, she inadvertently slipped up and the Professional Conduct Committee does not think it is right to pursue this, she is seen as being 'Let off' rather than a good professional who did what could happen to anyone. She belongs to a profession *which must never make a mistake*. Is this reasonable? Is this just? Is this right?

Reproduced with kind permission from Midwife, Health Visitor and Community Nurse, July/ August, Vol. 26, Nos. 7&8, 1990

Juno Lucina

The Association of Radical Midwives has petitioned the Lord Chancellor - as signatory of the Nurses, Midwives and Health Visitors (Professional Conduct) Rules 1987 Approval Order 1987, to ask him to look into the way these rules are being operated and whether changes are needed. The Association is concerned by what it sees as an apparent lack of awareness of the rules of natural justice in the carrying out of the Professional Conduct Machinery.

It is a scholarly and well researched document which has benefited from legal as well as midwifery input, and it has been sent to the Chairman of each of the national Boards. It suggests having a legally qualified chairman of the Professional Conduct Committee; it recommends that midwives should be judged by their peers; that accused midwives should be told the charges against them within three months, or the case dropped for want of prosecution; it wants the rules of evidence to be followed; and hearings of the Conduct Committee to be open to the public. The document criticises the length of sittings of the Professional Conduct Committee and points out that members of the panel adjudicating get too tired to concentrate if they are sitting listening for very long periods.

The document asks for the reasons behind decisions to be given, as is done in all other courts, and it suggests the use of intermediate penalties. Many of the suggestions are within the law as it now stands and it may just take a more detailed look at the laws under which the Conduct Committee and Investigating Committee operates for many of the suggestions to be taken on board.

The Association of Radical Midwives issued a document in 1986 called *The Vision - Proposals for the Future of the Maternity Services* and in this document proposed principles for good practice in the provision of maternity care, which would evolve from the principles that the relationship between the mother and the midwife is fundamentally important to good maternity care and that it is the mother who is the central person in the process of care. Their suggestions included women having realistic choices and that midwives skills should be fully utilised. The Association suggested continuity of care for all childbearing women and services based in the community. The service being accountable to those receiving care and that care should no harm to either mother or baby.

This far seeing vision of future maternity care has lent inspiration to many midwives, probably the vision of an improved professional conduct machinery will also inspire more midwives and help them to feel confident that they will get a fair hearing if they ever come before the Investigating Committee or the Professional Conduct Committee.

It would appear that this is what the midwife in 1989 wants and needs, especially at this moment when so many midwives feel demoralised and undervalued after the Clinical Grading which has appeared to denigrate the skills of the midwife and to fail to recognise either her expertise, her knowledge or the responsibility she takes. The midwife of 1989 wants and needs vision towards a positive future, strong leadership within the profession, and an assurance their she and her profession are really going somewhere. The profession is too demoralised at the moment for this impetus to come from within - it has to be led forward and both these documents pinpoint a better tomorrow for midwives and, because of the nature of the profession, for mothers.

Reproduced with kind permission from Midwives, Health Visitors and Community Nurse, March 1989.

Birthrights

*Caroline Flint reports on the impending threat to the personalized
midwifery care service in Hampshire*

In a sleepy corner of Hampshire women are up in arms, fighting for the maternity service which they have had for the past 20 years and taken for granted.

Women in Fairoak and Bishopstoke, near Winchester, had never realized that their maternity care was different from other women's – they just knew they liked it and enjoyed getting to know their two midwives, Jan Barnes and Sylvia Coles, who gave them antenatal care during their pregnancies.

When they went into labour they just telephoned whichever of the pair was on at the time.

After that either Jan or Sylvia came and looked after them in labour – either in their own home or, when the time was right, they all set off for the local general practitioner unit.

After the birth the two midwives visited the women daily to help a new mother to bath her new baby and change the nappy, or to discuss with experienced mothers good ways to incorporate the new baby into an existing family with as little jealousy as possible.

The women of Fairoaks and Bishopstoke have what they have been requesting for years – real continuity of care, where a familiar and trusted midwife provides care all the way through pregnancy, childbirth and the postnatal period. But now this excellent service is under threat.

The first blow came last October when the midwives were told that they were no longer allowed to claim for their overtime but in future would have to take time back 'in lieu'.

The midwives realized that this would be impossible because they work long and erratic hours, but because they love the job they carried on.

Soon another blow was to fall – they were told that in future they must not go out when not officially 'on call' and were threatened that if they did they would not be covered by the health authority's insurance protection.

Cathy McCormick, Royal College of Midwives' Senior Labour Relations Officer, is tackling this issue on two counts – first the disregard of 20 years of custom and practice, and second that legally employers cannot abrogate responsibility for the actions of their employees. Midwives, therefore, should always be covered by the health authority.

Vocal support

The midwives are also receiving support from a vocal group of local mums. Mandy Shedden, a mother of three, explained that the two midwives had given excellent and compassionate care over the years which women appreciated. But the health authority was suggesting that in future when a midwife is called to a woman in labour it has to be the midwife on call for the whole of the large area of Eastleigh – and that could be any one of eleven midwives unlikely to know the mother.

Mandy Shedden points out that as many of the other midwives come from miles away, they do not know the geography of the local area and may have problems finding the house. The other worry for the mothers is that many of the other midwives have not done a home birth for years out of preference.

As Mandy explains: 'Just imagine what it would be like having someone who didn't like home births sitting in your kitchen and you knew that she was the person looking after you during this crucial time in your in your life.'

The Capital Development Manager at the Royal Hampshire County Hospital Idwal Weale, said that although the midwives were working in line with 'patient demand', it was not in line with health authority policy which was to rationalize and streamline the provision of maternity care.

Senior midwife Ruth Nixon said that in Winchester they were not going for the principle of 'continuity of a known face' but for 'continuity of advice'.

The mothers are suspicious that the excellence of the care provided by their two local midwives is showing up the inadequacies of the rest of the service.

They have been told that the service can remain for a three month period while discussions take place. But they are worried that this is just a delaying tactic and that in three months' time a valuable service may have gone for ever.

Reproduced with kind permission from Nursing Standard, Vol. 4, No. 35, May 23 1990

Juno Lucina

Love is all you need, all you need is love says the song and I am beginning to think that a bit of it is what we need in midwifery today.

Midwives have grumbled (justifiably) at the takeover by obstetricians of childbirth, at the takeover by the computer giants such as Sony and Hewlett Packard who have made inestimable fortunes with electronic fetal monitors and ultrasound scanning equipment, while midwives have earned small salaries and worked long hours and actually 'done the work'. But now it is time to take stock.

Last year was a shameful year for midwives, not only because of the farce of the clinical grading review, but another more deep seated sore which was exposed, the torrent of accusation and blame which gripped our profession. With Jilly Rosser up before the Professional Conduct Committee, Caroline Flint up before the Investigating Committee, nearly all the independent midwives being questioned, supervised, investigated – no midwife who spoke out, no midwife who tried to be strong for women, felt safe.

Supervisors of midwives came under attack from the criticism levelled against them during the Rosser Case. The workings of the Professional Conduct Committee came under attack for the way it interpreted its own rules and conducted its business. As Juno looked down from Olympus at the goings-on in the world of midwifery she began to realize that what she was seeing was the tip of a very large iceberg, the blaming and accusation was actually rising up from the very bottom until it permeated all the way through this great and old profession.

Sometimes the blame and accusation was because the accuser herself lacked confidence and felt better if she could say 'Tut Tut, I don't approve of the way that midwife works, I would never do what she did.' Sometimes the accuser herself felt under threat so she pointed the finger at another colleague in the hope that the attention would be deflected from her.

An extraordinary psychology has evolved within the childbirth services – that is, that death is unwarranted and it has to be someone's fault. If a baby dies a perinatal meeting is called and everyone looks round on the person who can have the blame pinned on them – everyone who was off duty on the day in question heaves a sigh of relief, everyone who didn't deal with that woman feels justified and exonerated despite the fact that they were probably caring for the woman in the next room in a very similar way. As a result of a baby dying labour ward policies may be changed within an instant, something that has always been acceptable and unchallenged is now *verboten* and must never be done again. Our practice needs to be based on research and knowledge, not on over-emotional reactions. Everyone grieves when a baby dies, everyone is heart-broken when a mother dies, it is a terrible thing to happen and part of grief is to try and pin the blame on somebody or something, to ensure that life is controllable and to pretend to ourselves that if we always behave in a 'perfect' way we ourselves will be immortal.

Death is part of life, in the same way that laughing is, and being born and giving birth are. It is the feelings of panic and fear which permeate many labour wards which make the blaming and accusation a natural sequel. Often I identify the panic and fear as being fear of mortality itself; the flip side of this coin needs to be exposed in order to help the tension and accusing to flow away, the flip side of the coin is loving and cherishing.

Midwives need consciously to begin to love and support each other, and to consciously love and support obstetricians, in the same way that for every midwives have loved and supported women.

With love and cherishing of each other, we shall be able to stop blaming each other, just imagine the dreaded words 'Come to my office I want to talk to you about your conduct of Mrs Jones' delivery' – just imagine how much better that midwife would feel if with her she had eight other midwives who came along because they loved her and because they wanted to learn with her a better way of caring for the Mrs Joneses of this world.

Have you ever wondered how Jilly Rosser managed to survive her dreadful ordeal? It was love, love from mothers and love from other midwives and doctors who saw and recognized a midwife who cared about women and who was a woman of great integrity herself – love, it's all we need.

Reproduced with kind permission from Midwife, Health Visitor and Community Nurse, September 1989, Vol. 25, No. 9.

A Matter of Judgement

Independent midwife Jilly Rosser won her appeal in the High Court to be reinstated. But Caroline Flint argues midwives are still in a 'no win situation'

'We all make mistakes – even lawyers and doctors make mistakes, but we are not struck off for them'. So said Lord Justice Watkins in the case of Rosser versus the United Kingdom Central Council for Nursing, Midwifery and Health Visiting (UKCC), on Thursday, February 23, 1989.

On hearing these words, many of us in the court hoped that his judgement would include a definition of misconduct which would ensure that an injustice on the scale of that perpetrated against Jilly Rosser would never happen to a nurse, midwife or health visitor again. We were to be disappointed. Lord Justice Watkins was not to give a judgement because at the beginning of the second day of Rosser's appeal to the High Court the UKCC's barrister Mr James Badenoch conceded the case. He admitted that a serious irregularity had occurred when rebuttal evidence, which should have confined itself to specific matters, was used to cover the whole range of the Council's case.

The judge was not only critical of the misuse of the term 'misconduct', he also questioned the unrealistic expectations of midwives' capabilities. When discussing Jilly Rosser's alleged 'failure to keep accurate notes', the judge asked to see the notes, and read them. He suggested that they were satisfactory 'until the balloon went up' and at that time, he pointed out to Mr Badenoch, the midwife was busy examining the woman, telephoning the GP and the hospital and preparing for immediate transfer to hospital. The judge asked whether the council could realistically expect a midwife to be sitting down writing copious notes at the same time. The reply from Mr Badenoch caused titters in the court: he claimed that most midwives could be jotting down the notes while holding a mother's hand. The judge's robust reply was 'she would have to be a first class juggler'.

The judge indicated that the court was minded to find the charge against Rosser, that she had taken the woman to hospital in the back of a private car, perverse. He suggested that the charge was actually that she had not summoned the emergency services and that the charge about the private car was all part and parcel of the same charge. He also asked the Council's barrister what would have happened to Rosser if she had just waited for the emergency services 'Would she be in the same situation that she is in now?'

This helps to highlight the 'no win situation' many midwives are in – that whatever course they take, whatever decision they make, if those in authority over them decide to try and remove them, they can always find a case against the midwife.

Perhaps this vulnerability when taking clinical decisions is what has prompted the Association of Radical Midwives in its recent paper to the Lord Chancellor, *Professional Conduct Machinery for Midwives*[1] – *Some necessary changes* to suggest that: 'Unless it is clearly shown that clinical decisions were taken without reasonable assessment of the prevailing circumstances, a midwife's judgement in a particular situation should not be questioned by the Professional Conduct Committee.'

Lord Justice Watkins, with Mr Justice Phillips, allowed Jilly Rosser's appeal. They awarded costs against the UKCC, and the Professional Conduct Committee on September 10, 1988, was quashed – it is as if the charge had never been brought and that Jilly Rosser had never been struck-off as a midwife. But of course, the situation cannot really revert to what it was before the charge was brought. The fact that Jilly Rosser lost at least £15,000 in earnings is injustice enough, but if the UKCC does not act on this case and begin to put its house in order, the injustice will go on.

It is obvious that the UKCC capitulated because it was justifiably in fear of what would come out in the judgement; it was an exercise in damage limitation. But if it or any other body suggests that Jilly Rosser has been reinstated to the midwives' register because of a 'procedural irregularity' the injustice goes on.

The Professional Conduct Committee has always pointed out that it has a legal adviser sitting with it – the case of Rosser alone demonstrates that this is not safeguard enough. The Association of Radical Midwives in its document suggests that the Professional Conduct Committee should have a legally qualified chair – someone able to sift evidence, someone with experience of examining witnesses, reaching decisions, awarding penalties and interpreting the rules of procedure. This would help to assure an accused midwife that the committee will hear her evidence in an unbiased and unprejudiced way.

The Association of Radical Midwives also suggests that reasons for a decision should be given. No one to this day is entirely sure why Rosser was judged in the way that she was judged, because the Professional Conduct Committee does not have to give reasons for its decisions.

To be a member of a profession is both an honour and privilege. It carries weighty responsibility and to be in charge of the safety of mother and baby is an awesome responsibility. It is essential that midwives be ensured compassion and justice from those who sit in judgement on them.

•The UKCC was invited to reply to Caroline Flint's article, but declined.

Reference
1. The Association of Radical Midwives. (1989). *Professional Conduct Machinery for Midwives – Some Necessary Changes*

Reproduced with kind permission from Nursing Times, March 22, Volume 85, 1989.

Juno Lucina

Midwifery matters

What a strange and threatened group the midwifery profession is. Take the case of Jilly Rosser – brought to book after using her clinical judgement. One of a band of articulate and strong midwives deeply committed to taking their profession forward by increasing public and professional awareness of the profession by skilled use of, and a comfortable familiarity with the media.

Look at her case, and the treatment of any of the midwives who are using the media to promote midwives and midwifery to the public at large, and you will notice how these midwives are generally reviled, hounded and sorely criticized by their peers. In some cases their harassment goes as far as actual censorship by threatening them with, or actually carrying out, disciplinary measures.

We also need to be aware that one of the reasons for the unrest at present within the Royal College of Midwives is about that very issue – that the Royal College of Midwives is not getting enough publicity for its members. However, the two are not compatible. Midwives want their profession to be viewed comfortably by the media and to be able to use it for promotion of the role and practice of midwifery. This requires the realization that this can never be painfree and smooth, and that the important passage which one hoped would be immediately taken up by all the papers, was never quoted (and if it was quoted at all it would have been misquoted), and something quite banal and off the point was flashed across the nation for all to see. The media is not controllable although familiarity with its motions brings greater effectiveness, but whoever gets quoted will rarely be completely pleased with the article (nor with the photograph 'It's *terrible,* I don't look anything like that!').

As a group the midwifery profession has to realize that these are two sides of the same coin; you can't clip the wings of every midwife who is quoted in the local press or who writes something that you don't like and at the same time ask for more publicity for all matters related to midwifery. Either the profession recognizes its need for publicity or it remains permissible to say 'We like to hide our light under a bushel, we don't believe in broadcasting what we do to the world.' That attitude belongs in the Ark. Each and every midwife must take responsibility in informing the nation about their profession, and this means telling someone every day that they are midwives and what they actually do. It means actually writing down about what is happening in the ward or community or district and submitting it for publication and not leaving the writing of articles about midwifery to a tiny few.

The reason that the RCM members are so angry, want publicity and are threatening industrial action, is because of the treatment of midwives under the clinical grading review. It appears that most midwifery sisters are being offered 'F' grade on the scale which represents an increase of four per cent in their salary – less than inflation. So much for the government's cries about 'extra money for the nurses' and their support of those who carry on and never go on strike. Here is a profession which has never sanctioned strike action, which has kept its head down and carried on caring for the mothers and babies of the nation, promoting good health during pregnancy, delivering 76 per cent of the nation's babies. encouraging good mothering practices and what recognition does this sterling and uncomplaining work generate? None.

Perhaps the time has come when Ruth Ashton needs to be as recognized as Brenda Dean was. After all, the actions of her members have probably more impact on every member of the human race than the members of any union. But this recognition will not happen in a vacuum and midwives have to abandon their ambivalence towards the media and realize that this is how we communicate with each other and with our clients in the twentieth century. Yes, it is the time consuming, yes, it is hard work, and yes, it does involve *me* (I'm just an ordinary Staff Midwife after all) and *me* (I'm just an ordinary sister who doesn't want to rock the boat) and *me* (I'm a Midwifery Manager and from now on I shall encourage the midwives under me to speak out) - it involves every member of the profession. Is the profession up to it?

Reproduced with kind permission from Midwife, Health Visitors and Community Nurses, October 1988.

Discipline and Clinical Judgement

There seems to be a plethora of midwives being disciplined, suspended, reported - not by their patients, not by doctors, not by their peers but by their supervisors of midwives.

This one could say, is a perfectly satisfactory occurrence; midwives who are practising unsafely should be criticised, should be brought to task. No one wants a dangerous midwife to be working and attending women in labour and around childbirth - how true, but are the two synonymous?

Is it the unsafe midwife who is being disciplined? What is actually happening in this beleaguered profession?

All midwives have to comply with the Midwives Rules and the midwives' Code of Practice and all nurses, midwives and health visitors have to comply with the Code of Professional Conduct - all issued by the United Kingdom Central Council for Nurses, Midwives and Health Visitors.

The Midwives Rules are simple and uncontroversial. They demand of midwives a yearly notification of intention to practise and five yearly refresher courses: they show how midwives may be suspended from practice and they define a midwife's sphere of practice.

Dilemmas

The Code of Practice is equally wide and uncontroversial. It is usually easy to practise as a midwife and keep within the rules. But not always, sometimes there are dilemmas and sometimes there are instances where a clinical decision - looked at with the wisdom of hindsight - can be seen as questionable and that another decision could have been taken.

This is where the conflict arises since the difficulty for midwives is that their supervisors of midwives are not usually clinical practitioners. The clinical midwife therefore is being judged by someone who is not a clinician.

Most supervisors of midwives are managers, they have invariably been clinicians at some period of their life and probably were excellent when they were, which is probably why someone suggested they should climb up the ladder.

This does cause a great dilemma - clinical practice is what is happening now, today. It is not what happened three years ago, or even ten years ago, nor is it what happened twenty years ago. Clinical practice develops and changes, what was normal practice ten years ago would be seen as bizarre treatment today and even more so that which happened twenty years ago.

Other professions keep themselves clinically up to date by continuing to practise clinically. The solicitor who is the senior partner in a firm or the barrister who is head of chambers, the consultant obstetrician, the professor of medicine all practise and continue to practise, sometimes much less than their colleagues, but none the less they 'keep their hand in.'

In midwifery we have chosen another route and a route which we need to look at and question.

Management

In this profession clinical practice is often seen as a step on the ladder to management and that clinicians are less than their management colleagues. Sometimes this is true, but some clinicians choose to stay as clinicians and not become managers.

This choice guarantees a lower salary, lower status and judgement on their clinical practice by people who are not clinicians. This can cause great angst among midwives and is not beneficial to the profession as a whole. Every time a midwife is disciplined it intimidates those around her, it ripples through our profession and midwives feel under threat and vulnerable.

This only happens with local disciplinary hearings. Once the midwife is investigated by the investigating committee on the board she is judged by her peers - other practising midwives, other clinicians. This has to be much fairer but by the time her case gets there the midwife has suffered weeks of anxiety and worry, her confidence is shattered, she is intimidated and fearful.

Her case may or may not go on to the professional conduct committee of the UKCC and then she may be found guilty of misconduct. This misconduct can be a one off happening where a previously blameless midwife misjudges a situation. She can be struck off the register or it can be confirmed there was evidence of professional misconduct but the committee will take no action or will postpone judgement until a future date.

Unfairness

All these actions give the midwife little chance of defending her action in the light of what was happening at the time. The greatest unfairness of these hearings is that the midwife only has to slip up once.

With most practitioners, such as our medical colleagues, unless they have done something utterly crass, they have to show a pattern of poor clinical practice before they are chastised. With midwives it need only be a one off slip up.

Is this right? Is this useful to the profession? Is it useful to mothers and babies? Is the severity too great? I think so.

Reproduced with kind permission from Primary Health Care, November 1987

Conflicting Allegiances

Is a split developing in the midwifery hierarchy, and if so why? Caroline Flint explores two recent incidents which provide cause for concern

What is happening on the Isle of Wight where a community midwife was told that all patients must be given Syntometrine (see *Nursing Times* News, January 14, 1987) is only an echo of what is happening throughout the country where the midwife's right to practise her profession is increasingly coming under attack.

In a report in 1983, Robinson, Golden and Bradley[1] alerted us to the fact that in a third of all consultant obstetric units the decision over when to rupture membranes was made by unit policy and not by the midwife relating to the individual woman's needs. The decision to carry out vaginal examinations had nothing to do with the needs of the individual woman or the professional judgement of the midwife, but was unit policy in 50 per cent of consultant obstetric units.

Reviewing the report, Pat Ferguson said, 'The doctors, particularly the junior staff, see midwives as advisers rather than clinicians' and added, 'it seems clear that the UK will shortly have an American-style system of obstetric nursing, rather than the high-status midwifery practised in the rest of Europe'[2].

In response to instructions that Syntometrine must be given to all patients, Royal College of Midwives general secretary Ruth Ashton said, 'Our organization does not support any umbrella policies which take away the proper clinical judgement opportunities of anyone.' This underlines the Midwife's Code of Practice which states that, 'each midwife as a practitioner is accountable for her own practice in whatever environment she practises'.[3]

This attitude also reflects midwifery in the same light as the World Health Organization's definition of the midwife, adopted in 1972 by the International Federation of Gynaecologists and Obstetricians. This states that, 'a midwife ... must be able to give the necessary supervision, care and advice to women during pregnancy, labour and the postpartum period, to conduct deliveries on *her own responsibility* and to care for the newborn and the infant.'

The case about using Syntometrine came to light in the same week that I heard of an area where community midwives who stay on call voluntarily for women booked for a domino delivery, have also received notice that, 'Midwives are not allowed to visit any patients in labour at home unless they are the midwife on call that day.'

Midwives' practice is being attacked on several fronts and who is responsible? The consultants? They are up to a point because to increase their own sphere of practice necessitates restricting the midwife's, but even more the attack is coming from senior midwives. They do not seem to ally themselves with their own profession but with the obstetricians – which is a direct result, I would suggest, of the hierarchical way in which we have arranged our profession. The effect is that the most senior midwives become isolated both from their fellow midwives and the women they care for, and in their loneliness turn to the only other group with which they have contact – the obstetricians.

So what should the senior midwife on the Isle of Wight have done when she was asked by a consultant to tell the midwife in question to use Syntometrine? Ideally, she should have refused and pointed out that this was a matter for the midwife's professional judgement. At the least, she should have agreed to say that the consultant 'recommended' the use of Syntometrine, but she should certainly not have issued an instruction to say that all women were to receive it. It is pleasing to learn that the health authority has now effectively acknowledged this point. (see *News*, p.8)

Likewise, what is the senior midwife in the case of domino deliveries thinking of when trying to change the established practice of midwives, which is obviously very much for the benefit of the women they are caring for? If midwives have been in the practice of seeing women in early labour at home even though the midwife herself is not on call, that practice cannot be changed without proper consultation. If the midwives refuse to change this practice because they believe that it is beneficial for women then nothing can be done about it.

The employer should be leaping up and down with joy that he employs people who are so committed that they are willing to go beyond the call of duty. This is expected of all professionals. The only obligation of the midwife who has been up all night is that she must be in a fit and proper condition to do her work when she is supposed to be on duty and this is her decision, not her employers. She can be challenged by her employer only if it is patently obvious that the midwife is not in a fit and proper condition.

As for the old chestnut that 'You're not covered when you aren't on duty' – as a professional you are responsible for your own practice, so it is essential that you are covered by indemnity insurance either with the RCM or with one of the trade unions.

And to lonely midwife managers I would say, whatever you do affects us and ultimately the women we care for. You are in the difficult position of being the spearhead for midwifery, you must support our profession. It is you who can make or break us.

References
1. Robinson, S., Golden, J., Bradley, S. (1983). *A study of the role and responsibilities of the midwife.* London: DHSS.
2. Ferguson, P. (1984). 'Midwifery under threat.' *Senior Nurse*; Vol 1, p.27.
3. UKCC (1986). *A Midwife's Code of Practice for Midwives Practising in the United Kingdom.* London: UKCC.
4. Klein, M., Lloyd, I., Redman, C., Bull, M., Turnbull, A. (1983). 'A comparison of low-risk pregnant women booked for delivery in two systems of care: shared-care (consultant) and integrated general practice unit.' *British Journal of Obstetrics and Gynaecology* : Vol. 90: 2, pp.118-128.

Reproduced with kind permission from Nursing Times, February 4, 1987.

Midwives' Judgement

Recent events in the Isle of Wight suggest that midwives are being hampered in their role as practitioners and their right to use their clinical judgement. Caroline Flint argues that midwives are clinicians and that unless they are practising dangerously they must not be beholden to uniform directives from obstetricians

The row in the Isle of Wight over the right of midwives to use their professional judgement[1], is not over. It is, however, heartening to read that the senior midwife involved has the support of her colleagues, as letters to this week's correspondence columns show.

I'm so glad to hear that if they were not in agreement with unit policy these midwives would feel free to discuss their views with their nursing officer/ supervisor of midwives and obstetricians and that they feel confident their views would be given every consideration. It is the right of all employees throughout the land to have their views heard by their employer in relation to their work and conditions of service and to expect those views to be given every consideration.

But these midwives appear to have missed the point of what this rumpus is all about – unlike the 29 people who have written to Mary Cronk to pledge their support and to tell her of yet more awful examples. They have recognized that this is about a practitioner's right to practise.

A midwife is a practitioner, wherever she works. This is underlined in the World Health Organization's definition of a midwife: 'A midwife ... must be able to give the necessary supervision, care and advice to women during pregnancy, labour and the postnatal period, to conduct deliveries *on her own responsibility* and to care for the newborn and the infant' (my italics).

The status of a practitioner is different from any other employee in that a practitioner *practises* and uses her clinical judgement.

What is happening throughout the country is that 'unit policies' are being drawn up with defined clinical actions, and midwives are being expected to follow them unquestioningly. If they are employed as obstetric nurses with responsibility to the obstetricians, they can follow the policies quite happily. But if they are employed as midwives this is impossible for them to do; as midwives their responsibility is to provide the best care possible to that particular mother and baby. And this cannot be carried out with uniform policies because no woman is the same as any other woman, and, equally, no labour and no baby are the same as any other. So it needs clinical judgement on the part of the midwife to ensure that this mother and baby receive the best, the safest and the most supportive care appropriate to their needs; it cannot be pre-determined.

This is not to say that guidelines cannot be written; for instance 'Mr Rogers recommends that all his patients should be accelerated with Syntocinon if their cervix does not dilate at the rate of one centimetre an hour once labour is established' a guideline based on O'Driscoll and Meagher[2]; or 'The supervisor of midwives suggests that all women who wish to breastfeed should be encouraged to put the baby to the breast within an hour of delivery and frequently (at least every two hours) for the first 24 hours following delivery)' as Salariya et al.[3] suggest; or 'Miss Jones recommends the artificial rupture of membranes when the cervix of any of her patients reaches four-five centimetres in order to assess fetal condition' as quoted by O'Driscoll and Meagher[2].

These recommendations and suggestions may be relevant for this particular woman. But then again, they may not.

For example, the midwife has a woman in labour who is a patient of Miss Jones. The woman's labour is progressing well, the baby's heartbeat is strong and firm and regular and the midwife decides in this instance that artificial rupture of the membranes is inappropriate. When questioned she refers to Dunn on the hazards and disadvantages of amniotomy and the increase in perinatal mortality following its use, quoted in the *Proceedings* of the *Sixth European Congress on Perinatal Medicine in Vienna*[4] and the World Health Organization' recommendation that 'artificial early rupture of membranes, as a routine process, is not justifiable'[5]. In her clinical judgement at this time artificial rupture of membranes is not appropriate for this woman. In retrospect she may regret this decision; there may be some reason why she wished she had ruptured the membranes earlier, but this is irrelevant. To quote O'Driscoll[2]: 'Medicine in real life does not include the luxury of wisdom after the event'. It is the duty of the midwife to do *at the time*, what she considers best in her clinical judgement. And because of this she cannot follow a prescribed route. This is the reason that no midwife can be told: 'always give Syntometrine' or 'always rupture membranes' or 'always use electronic fetal monitoring'.

The midwife is a clinician and a practitioner in the same way as a doctor is. The only difference is that the midwife's sphere is limited to normal childbirth, whereas the doctor's ranges over the whole field of medicine.

The safety of the women in a midwife's care is safeguarded by the role of the supervisor of midwives. If the midwife is practising dangerously or not in accordance with the Midwives' Rules, the supervisor of midwives may then – and only then – intervene to check her practice. She cannot intervene merely because, in the exercise of her own clinical judgement, she would have done something differently.

References

1. 'Midwife wins clinical judgement battle' (News). *Nursing Times*. (1987). 83: 5,8.
2. O'Driscoll, K., Meagher, D. (1980). *Active Management of Labour.* London: W. B. Saunders Co.
3. Salariya, E.M., Easton, P.M., Cater, J.I. (1978). 'Duration of breastfeeding after early initiation and frequent feeding.' *The Lancet* ; 2: 8100, pp.1141-3.
4. Dunn, P.M. In: George Thieme (1979). *Proceedings of the Sixth European Congress on Perinatal Medicine, Vienna, 1978.* Stuttgart.
5. World Health Organization. (1985). *Appropriate Technology for Birth.* Geneva: WHO.

Reproduced with kind permission from Nursing Times, March 4, 1987.

Trouble and Strife

Conflict within the midwifery profession is rearing its ugly head. Caroline Flint calls for more discussion as a means of averting disciplinary action

A midwife delivers a stillborn baby to a woman she has become very close to - the baby obviously died 12 hours prior to the onset of labour with *placenta abruptio*. During the night which follows the anguished midwife stays and comforts the mother, sharing her grief, giving comfort and solace. The husband, in his anguish, says that he is going to sue. He wants an inquiry; he wants to complain. Who can he sue? God? The world? Life? The Tory Party?

The next morning the midwife is suspended from duty and practice, leaving the mother not only grieving but now feeling terribly guilty about her midwife. Were her husband's ravings the cause of her midwife's suspension?

A vocal midwife, strong in her profession, a hard worker delivering mothers at home and in hospital with commitment and kindness, is a by-word with the mothers in her district, having delivered many others of several children. Known and respected by her local GPs, relied upon by younger colleagues for advice and support and for her professional expertise, whose paper work has never been her first priority, the midwife is challenged by her supervisor over her treatment of a woman during the first stage of labour. The supervisor cautions her about her note-keeping and insists that she work in the antenatal clinic under the supervision of a much less experienced midwife (one who doesn't get up the supervisor's nose so much). The midwife can't bear it and slinks away, like a criminal, to work in a medical ward - lost to midwifery for ever. Did any women complain about her care? No. Did any GP complain

about her care? No. Was there any query about her competence? No, but it's easy to destroy a midwife.

An articulate midwife is summoned to meetings with her senior midwives almost every month. She runs active birth classes and encourages women to make out birth plans, which some midwives in her unit find threatening. She starts to become suspicious about these 'informal' meetings when she notices that her personnel file is getting bigger and bigger. One day she delivers a baby and it has to go to the special care baby unit. Another 'informal' meeting is arranged, this time with a paediatrician and an obstetrician and both her senior midwives. The midwife decides to take a colleague with her as she is beginning to feel outnumbered. The midwife is not allowed to go into the meeting with her colleague and the meeting takes place without her. The next day she is summoned to a disciplinary hearing for being in breach of her contract because she refused to attend meetings with her seniors!

What is Caroline ranting on about, you might be saying. She has been listening to the demented outpourings of aggrieved midwives. She has only heard one side of each of these cases. I also thought that might be the case, until I received this letter in the post:

'After I took out a grievance following an attempt to change my contracted hours I was subjected to almost constant victimization and harassment. While working in the labour ward I would suddenly be sent somewhere else because they were busy there. This began to happen two out of every three days I was working. I had constant meetings with senior midwives with no complaints about my work, but complaints about my record-keeping (and as I'm very articulate and write well, I felt that this was just an excuse). Finally, things came to a head when the senior midwife called me into her office and told me that I would be disciplined for some travel expense errors paid to me over 12 months previously. In despair, having had support but little expertise from RCM and RCN stewards, I contacted a solicitor who managed to come to a disciplinary meeting held on a Sunday after two days' notice. I was suspended from duty and was given a final written warning, which was better than the dismissal which my director of midwifery services wanted - the finance department had paid me in error an extra £8. I keep applying to do my advanced diploma of midwifery or an ultrasound course, but I am not being allowed study leave. How can midwives be so cruel to each other?'

How can we be so cruel to each other? I keep getting letters from community midwives who have always stayed 'on call' for women they wanted to deliver and who are now being refused permission to do this. The reason given is that these women shouldn't be getting privileged treatment, that it is depriving other midwives of the opportunity to deliver babies. But since the other midwives have not been booking women for deliveries, they obviously haven't wanted to deliver. So midwives who want to provide a personalised service to women are not being allowed to.

Last week a woman told me that even though she was having a home delivery, she had been told she could have any one of 18 midwives to look after her when she goes into labour. Is this progress?

I have given these horrific examples which have all happened in different parts of the country during the past year.

The intelligent articulate, troublesome midwife is the flower of our profession. On her rests the hopes of women and midwives in this country. It is she who needs encouraging, helping and supporting. The midwife who is obedient and no trouble is not good news. Before your senior midwives discipline or threaten, count to 10 - no, 100 - and make sure that you are not doing it because of your own feelings of insecurity. Martyrs are not what the profession needs. We need strong, articulate and - yes - troublesome midwives.

Reproduced with kind permission from Nursing Times, November 6, 1985

Homebirth

These articles are Caroline's bid to convey to unbelievers the reasons why homebirth is such a worthwhile cause. The arguments put forward relate to cost, safety, client preference, intervention rates, midwifery autonomy, rest and sleep, family cohesion, convenience, privacy, social cohesion, tradition, job satisfaction, continuity of care, comfort and better mothering! These arguments, in various configurations, appeared in a range of publications – the National Childbirth Trust's *'New Generation'*, *Primary Health Care, Nursing Times, Socialism and Health, Nursing* and the *Journal of Obstetrics and Gynaecology*. The articles therefore represent a remarkable attempt to expose a considerable number of people to pro-homebirth propaganda and to sow seeds of doubt about the supremacy of hospital birth. As such it is reasonable to conclude that they have played a part in halting the decline of homebirth.

No opportunity to acquaint readers with Caroline's favourite articles and reports is lost. The work of Damstra-Wijmenga, Klein, Campbell and MacFarlane, Caldeyro-Barcia, Tew and Dunn are presented in numerous articles in this as in preceding sections. Their findings and conclusions, challenging as they do the dominant medical culture of childbirth, are not allowed to pass unheeded or sink without at least making impact on Caroline's readers.

Similarly the Royal College of Midwives' report 'Towards a Healthy Nation' is promoted in a number of these articles, despite the fact that its failure to adopt continuity of care as a central theme for the development of the maternity services must have been a frustration and disappointment for Caroline, who was a RCM Council member at the time. This rather bland report was published a year after the Association of Radical Midwives brought out its more foresighted 'Vision' for the future of the maternity services. However Caroline dwells on the aspect of 'Towards a Healthy Nation' that she found most positive, namely its endorsement of homebirth.

'A very special birth day' and 'No place like home for labour' both contain case studies of childbirth as it should be in Caroline's view: woman-centred, quiet and private and against a background of family and community life. The former article is also a quick guide on how to attend a birth as an independent midwife whilst working for the NHS. Caroline was not quite the innocent she makes out in this article or in 'Home service'. She is publicly retracing the origins of her own thinking and practice as a midwife for those coming after her. The three years break in attending any homebirths that she mentions in 'A very special birthday' was a purgatorial blip in a career which has centred on attending women giving birth in their own homes.

Caroline subscribes to the widely, but no means universally, shared view that the culture of birth underpins the ethos of society and that our experience of our own birth echoes throughout our lives. In 'Retracing our cultural roots', the far-reaching and cross-generational implications of our management of childbirth are outlined. The idea that the mode of giving birth can be imprinted on coming generations means that the way we approach birth has long lasting effects. The possibility that this is indeed likely is attested to by the theory of morphic resonance proposed in 'New Science' (Sheldrake, 1990). Caroline constantly asks her readers to consider what sort of society they want, what sort of people do we want to be and with what kinds of memories? Do we want to subject ourselves and our babies to technocratic management and thereby change something of who and what we are?

In 'Labour – the importance for a woman to be in control of her own childbearing' Caroline argues that control, choice and being enabled to take responsibility for oneself and one's loved ones are an essential part of being human and therefore a necessary foundation for maternity care. The rightness of homebirth for women, babies and families, as illustrated in 'A very special birthday', therefore prefigures the statistical support for its safeness. For proponents of homebirth like Caroline, the findings of Tew, and Campbell and MacFarlane were no more surprising than spring being followed by summer. The fact nonetheless re-mains that, for many midwives, doctors and women, the exhortation to homebirth is more akin to being invited on a round-the -world cruise in medieval times, when it was well known that the Earth was flat.

In 1990, Caroline and Valerie Taylor set up their 'Special Delivery Midwifery Practice' as outlined in the article of that title. They made a deliberate and conscious decision to attract influencial people as their clients in the belief that such clients, traditionally the private patients of obstetricians, could really help to bring about a change in the public's perception of homebirth and midwifery. As a result they have to brook a lot of criticism from other midwives that what they are doing somehow isn't really proper midwifery, an accusation they strongly refute. Meanwhile the practice has thrived and, in 1994, they opened their Birth Centre, the first free-standing independent birth centre in the UK, in Tooting, South London.

Reference
Sheldrake, R. (1990). *The Rebirth of Nature: New Science and the Revival of Animism*. London: Rider Books.

Why GPs Should Back Home Births

By Caroline Flint, midwifery sister at St George's Hospital, Tooting

A month ago I booked a woman for a home delivery for her second child who is due next March. I wrote to her GP to inform him that I had booked her and that she would be cancelling her hospital booking. I also asked him if he would be willing to provide medical cover for the delivery, but if he was unwilling to do this I would arrange with the local supervisor of midwives to transfer the patient to the local obstetric unit in the case of any abnormality arising. I also asked the GP if he wished to continue with shared antenatal care with me instead of the hospital.

Having treated the doctor in a professional and polite way, I received no reply to my letter. I then also heard from the patient that when she went to see the GP he tried to frighten her about having a baby at home - quoting instances about seeing women bleed to death at home and telling her about the risks and dangers of home birth. All this to a Gravida two, well nourished, well educated, non smoking woman with suitable housing, whom I delivered of her first child two years ago. The whole pregnancy, labour and puerperium could not have been more normal.

Continuum

I have not yet met this GP. I am used to working with GPs who are supportive to women and who see themselves as providing a continuum of care which spans the whole family and the whole of life from birth to death. It seems to me that this GP is not only letting down his patient but also his profession. If GPs are not willing to provide a service which women are asking for - I suggest they will lose out eventually.

The reason I see the GP losing out eventually is because, as a midwife, I don't need him. I am qualified to look after a woman throughout a normal pregnancy, labour and the puerperium and I only need to refer to a doctor 'should any illness or abnormality of the woman, fetus or baby become apparent.' The doctor I refer to does not have to be the woman's GP, it can be the obstetric registrar on call at the local maternity unit, and this would probably be far more appropriate.

The other reason I see the GP losing out is that it seems to be more and more difficult for a GP to provide maternity care within the hospital. With the increased closure of GP maternity beds and with the new, more stringent requirements to get on the obstetric list I can see the GP disappearing from full maternity care and only able to provide a minimal antenatal service together with his community midwife.

So what shall I do about this GP? Shall I leave him alone and let him go on frightening pregnant women? Or shall I send him the paper by Rona Campbell and others?[1] They looked at every birth which took place at home in 1979 and they discovered that when a baby was born to a woman who was unbooked, the perinatal mortality rate was 196.9/1000. The perinatal mortality rate for a woman who was booked for a hospital delivery but actually delivered at home was 67.5/1000, but the perinatal mortality rate for women booked for a home delivery was 4.1/1000.

High risk

Shall I send one by Damstra-Wijmenga MD[2] who looked at all the women in Groningen in Holland who had babies in 1981. A table of 1,692 women took part in his survey, of these 11.7 per cent had no choice as to where to deliver, they were women who we would term 'high risk' and they were referred to an obstetrician and had their care in hospital. The rest of the women had a choice: they could deliver at home; they could deliver in hospital and stay for just 24 hours; or they could deliver in hospital and stay for a week.

Damstra-Wijmenga shows that 'among those women who had opted for home confinement significantly fewer complications occurred during pregnancy, delivery and puerperium than among those who had their babies in hospital followed by a 24-hour stay there or followed by a seven-day stay in a maternity ward. Morbidity was also lower among the babies born at home than among those born in hospital.'

He surmises, 'for a normal healthy woman after a pregnancy without complication, it is questionable whether a hospital is, in fact, the "safer" place for having a baby. It should be realized that when a woman decides to have her baby in an environment designed to cope with childbirths in which there is a certain degree of risk, there is a good chance that the hospital facilities will actually be used on her, thus imposing a risk of iatrogenic damage.'

It is obvious that home confinements are safe for low risk women who are booked with a midwife for a home birth. I wonder, therefore, if my GP points out any of the dangers of hospital delivery to the women who book with him - increased risk of infection, increased risk of intervention, increased risk of separation of mother and baby, interruption in family life with the father being excluded during the postnatal period. It is naive to believe that just by being inside a hospital all risks melt away.

References

1. Campbell R. 'Home Births in England and Wales, 1979: perinatal mortality according to intended place of delivery.' *British Medical Journal* 1984, 289: pp.721-724.
2. Damstra-Wijmenga S. 'Home Confinement: the positive results in Holland.' *Journal of the Royal College of General Practitioners*, August 1984, pp. 425-30.

Reproduced with kind permission from Primary Health Care, January 1986.

A Very Special Birth Day

Being asked to deliver a friend's baby at home is an incredible honour, writes Caroline Flint. There is a lot to do but the atmosphere surrounding the birth makes everything worthwhile

Becky rang. 'Caroline, I'm expecting another baby on October 3. I want to have it at home, will you deliver me?'

'Becky, I can't. I work full time in the health service and you live outside my health district. How can I?'

'But I want to.'

I hadn't seen a home delivery for three years and I needed to. How could I attempt to make hospital more 'home-like' if I hadn't been at a home birth for so long? Really, I needed to do it. For my own professional development I needed to be involved in a home birth again.

And what an honour was being bestowed on me. I was being asked to be involved in one of the most important moments in my friend's life; one of the most intimate, one of the most exciting. How could I refuse? Especially when I wanted to do it so much?

So my first answer to Becky was yes, but then I had to go through the mechanics of delivering a friend at home.

First, I booked a fortnight's holiday.

Second, I wrote to the supervisor of midwives of Becky's district and explained what I intended to do and I asked her for an intention to practise form. Later I asked her for a birth notification form and a Guthrie test form. I had then fulfilled my legal requirements.

Third, I contacted another midwife who practises independently and asked her if she would act as a my 'cover' in case I should break my leg. She agreed and, in the event, acted as my photographer.

Fourth, I went to see my own supervisor of midwives and explained that I intended to do this home delivery in my holiday. She was very kind. Although she is not very keen on home deliveries she offered to lend me the equipment I would need as long as I filled in the labour ward borrowing book. This I gladly agreed to do.

What if I hadn't been so fortunate in my own supervisor? Perhaps the supervisor in Becky's district would have allowed me to borrow the appropriate equipment; the role of the supervisor is, after all, to give support to the midwives practising in her area.

If I had had to buy all the equipment I needed it would have cost me £200-£250. This would buy a stethoscope, sphygmomanometer, Pinard's stethoscope, two pairs of large Spencer Wells forceps, scissors, plain or toothed dissecting forceps, stitch holder, stainless steel receiver to boil them all up in, sterile gloves, baby resuscitation bag and mask, sterile sutures and mucus extractors and a packet of incontinence pads. If I'd wanted to add gilt to the gingerbread I could also have bought a portable sonicaid for approximately £320.

Syntometrine can be supplied by a local chemist but he or she will need proof that you are a qualified midwife and usually they will take a day or two to obtain the ampoules. They will also sell you the equipment to give the Synometrine.

If they are unsure about issuing the Synometrine, refer them to Schedule IV Part III of the Medicines (Prescription Only) Order, 1980 and the Medicines Act 1968 (Part III).

When Becky first booked with me she had a GP who was willing to support her in having her baby at home. Sadly, during her pregnancy he became ill and wrote to her to say that he was sorry but he wouldn't be able to provide medical cover for her. I wrote to the local supervisor of midwives and let her know about this and said that if anything untoward occurred during Becky's pregnancy or labour I would get in touch with the local maternity unit if anything cropped up which necessitated medical care.

My first duty, according to the Midwives' Code of Practice, was to take a full history from Becky as soon as practicable. I bought a firm exercise book and took a very full history of her physical, psychological and social needs, her past obstetric history, menstrual history, family medical history and history of this pregnancy. I must keep these records for ever and they must be available for the local supervisor of midwives to inspect. I must also send for a Register of Cases II from Hymns Ancient and Modern Ltd. It is nice for all midwives to have their own register of the women they have delivered and this is a useful way for a midwife to keep statistics of her practice .

Having fulfilled my legal obligations I continued with Becky's antenatal care and early one day after I had been on holiday for a week, the telephone rang. It was Becky.

'What are you planning to do Caroline?'

'Why? Are you in labour?'

'No, I just wanted to know, just in case. I've had a show, but nothing else is happening.'

I decided then that what I was doing was spending the day with Becky. I didn't want to miss any of the labour.

After a cup of coffee and a chat, I examined Becky and found her temperature, pulse, blood pressure and urine were normal. The baby's head was engaged and was lying in the right occipito-anterior position and his heart was beating regularly at 128 a minute. Becky's cervix was posterior, soft and thick and not dilated. She was having vague contractions which didn't seem either regular or very strong, but Becky was sure that she was in early labour.

The time was now 9.30am and Becky's other three children were beginning to appear. Her husband, Adrian, was due at a rehearsal and wondered whether to go or not. Becky assured him that he could. We sat and ate breakfast and helped the smaller children to dress.

The morning began to slip by pleasantly. At about 11.00am Becky said 'I meant to plant some wallflowers before this baby came. I'm going to nip to the garden centre and buy some.' I got up to accompany her but no, she wanted to go on her own and I was to stay and keep an eye on the other children. Towards midday I organized some lunch for them and began to worry about where Becky was - surely she must have got the wallflower plants by now? I didn't even know where the garden centre was.

Becky finally arrived home with two strange men (and her wallflower plants) an hour later. Her car had broken down and when she told her sad tale to the men at the garden centre they had offered to ring for an ambulance to take her to hospital. When she said that she was having her baby at home they nearly freaked out! They shut the garden centre and both came to give each other moral support!

Now it was time to check Becky and her baby again and time for the other children to go and play with friends up the road. Adrian arrived home from his rehearsal and quickly vacuumed the bedroom floor. Next he tacked a vast sheet of polythene to the floor and then a sheet on top of that. Becky was active, and mainly on her hands and knees at this stage; she flung off her clothes one by one as she became hotter until eventually she was naked. Adrian sat on the bed and munched a doorstep of bread and peanut butter. When he had finished he supported Becky in a semi-squat, and she rested comfortably on my Victorian porcelain bedpan, leaning against Adrian's knees as he sat on a pouffe. Then at 2.45pm Becky's membranes ruptured spontaneously, with clear liquor draining and once again my trusty bedpan came into its own and caught all the drips. (It was my grandmother's and I used it for all my labours.) I did my second vaginal examination of the labour (to exclude a prolapsed cord) and found Becky to be six centimetres dilated with a very thin cervix which was well applied to the head which was just above the level of the ischial spines. The baby's heart was beating regularly at 128 a minute.

The contractions were coming thick and fast now. Becky was standing, squatting, gyrating her pelvis, on all fours. Adrian was massaging her back, Nicky, the other midwife was taking photos and I was keeping my hands clean with a bowl of water in the corner and listening to the baby's heart.

Becky was calm, contented and relaxed. There was total silence in the room except for the occasional sighs and groans Becky made at the end of each contraction. The atmosphere was peaceful, almost sacramental, beautiful, full of anticipation. Another half hour passed, and Becky began to feel the urge to push and started doing so. I could see no external signs of full dilation and felt that I ought to make sure that Becky was really fully dilated. In fact she was still only 8cm but the head had descended further. The baby's heartbeat was strong and regular at 128 a minute.

We all encouraged Becky to pant instead of push, and she rested on her knees with her bottom in the air to help the urge to push. She managed well. More time passed; Becky took gulps of water between contractions. Fifteen minutes later the pushing urge became overwhelming and there were external signs of full dilation.

Becky was on her hand and knees, with Adrian at her side, and her friend Pauline at the edge of the tacked down sheet. The baby's little dark head edged its way out of the vagina. Because of the position, mucus ran out of his nose and mouth and was gently wiped away. The baby's body slipped out and I passed him up to his mother. It was Samuel. He gave a little whimper and then opened his eyes and gazed about him in amazement and with a puzzled expression, especially as the phone began to ring! I answered and spoke to Adrian's father and told him that he had another grandson but that we were all a bit busy and could he ring back in half-an-hour.

Pauline had by now rushed to get the other children. Becky was comfortably ensconced on the bedpan awaiting the arrival of the placenta while the baby was vigorously sucking. The children had by now all excitedly gathered round and Becky was busy ringing her mother to tell her the news. The placenta plopped out after half-an-hour, plus 400ml of blood. Becky's uterus was well contracted but she felt a little shaky and so was put to bed.

I had taken my kitchen scales to weigh the baby and he was seven pounds and three ounces. His Apgar score had been ten and he was a beautiful, alert baby. I clamped his cord and gently bathed him so that all the children could 'help'.

Becky had perked up again by now. She wriggled down to the end of the bed and I sat on the pouffe and sutured her small first degree tear, after which she decided to have a bath. I ran it for her and helped her in and out. After it, she went to the lavatory and passed urine.

My husband then arrived to take me out to dinner by which time, Becky, clean and warm, was lying in bed with Samuel snuggled beside her. He waited downstairs and was rather put out when a neighbour asked him if he was the grandfather!

After our dinner I went back to settle Becky down for the night. She was lying in bed watching the television, having had a lovely supper. Baby Samuel had passed meconium so I changed his nappy. Becky's uterus was well contracted and her lochia was not excessive. She had passed more urine and had my telephone number in case of any worries during the night. I was given a key for the morning as I would be very early and had offered to wake them with a cup of tea.

In the morning as I entered the room where Samuel had been born and I looked at his mother snuggled in bed next to Adrian, I anticipated the next few days when she would be petted and spoiled; queen of the household, the whole world revolving around her and baby Samuel. I thought that this is how it was meant to be - a woman surrounded by love, in her own home, part of the community around her but also very special. It had been a real birth day.

Reproduced with kind permission from Nursing Times, January 15 1986

Custom-built Birth At Home

I delivered a baby at home yesterday, for the first time in almost a year. All the babies I have delivered in the past eleven months have been born in hospital and almost nearly all the women I have looked after in labour have moved around a great deal in labour. Many have spent hours on end in the bath, many have used entonox, most have ended up by delivering in positions other than on a bed and lying down - on their hands and knees, standing up, on a birth chair, on their side or even in the bath.

Being privileged to be with women in labour has shown me the great diversity of the human spirit, the love and affection between a woman and her lover, the excitement of seeing a baby emerging, the pain, the joy, the strength, and the beauty of the human body working at its best.

During the labour at home I sometimes thought about being with women in labour in hospital and there were some things I really missed - the space primarily. The bedroom was much smaller than the delivery rooms in our hospital and the labouring woman had far less room to roam around in than she had when she had her first baby in hospital.

The second thing I really missed were the rubber mats which we have for our floors. They are truly marvellous and really comfortable for pregnant women to crawl on, lie on or sit on; they are also waterproof so that a clean sheet on top of them is the only equipment needed to ensure that the area is clean.

Those were the things I missed. What did I not miss? What was better about delivering a woman at home? First the equipment was all there, I had everything I needed inside the room or just outside the door. I knew I had everything I needed because I pack my own bag ready for home deliveries and it is my responsibility and mine alone to ensure that I have everything.

I didn't reach out for a thermometer, only to find it not there and have to say to Janie 'I've just got to pop and get a thermometer', or 'I've just got to go and get a spygmomanometer, I won't be long'. Or the syntometrine, or the vaginal examination trolley, or an extra pillow, or the resuscitaire, or a bottle of lotion, or a monitor or some more inco pads.

Privacy

The other thing that I really appreciated about delivering Janie at home was the privacy. It was her bedroom, in her house; when she looked up there were no prying eyes gazing in at her through a grille in the door. No-one burst into the room to 'borrow a sphyg' or to ask 'have you got a spare monitor?" No doctors came in to ask why I hadn't ruptured the membranes even though she was eight centimetres.

No one was there to cast any doubts on her ability to handle this situation, no anaesthetist came into to ask her what analgesia she had thought about. In fact the whole labour was conducted in peace and quiet as Janie's husband held her hand and whispered occasional encouraging words. I just sat and waited and listened to the fetal heart occasionally.

Janie's mother was there looking after their little son who I delivered three yeas previously, and whenever I put my head out of the bedroom door to ask for three cups of tea or coffee, they arrived in seconds. Soon Janie's parents-in-law also arrived and throughout the house there was an atmosphere of waiting, caring, thinking of Janie and only her. She was uppermost in everyone's minds, the house was filled with love and concern - everyone was rooting for her.

When Danielle arrived it was into a silent room, into warm and loving arms and into tranquil lighting. Within a few minutes she was looking around wondering where she had come to and then she decided she had come for a good meal and latched on.

It was after the birth that I remembered again what the great beauty of a home delivery is. By now Janie was in bed and Danielle had been inspected by grandparents and big brother, I had scooped all the newspapers and inco pads protecting the floor into a large black polythene bag (and the placenta well wrapped) and I had filled in my notes, register and birth notification. The household ticked on, the birth of this little person had happened and now everyone was getting on with preparing the lunch - the baby had been absorbed into the continuum of life.

Big brother came up to see his mother every now and then, but finding her rather boring because she was in bed and not ready to play, he went downstairs again, Janie sat in bed like a queen - eating a huge steak and drinking a large glass of red wine. She looked relaxed and content and very, very clever. Her husband was tired - he had been up all night and he lay beside her, snoozing in his own bed, next to his beloved woman who he had cherished and supported and next to his baby. He wasn't cut out, sent home, excluded.

Contentment

Today when I went in to see Janie the feeling had not changed. She was lying in bed and the television had been brought upstairs for her to watch. She lay in bed with her baby snuggled on one side sucking contentedly and her little son snuggled on the other side watching 'Thomas the Tank' with his mother.

The whole house is organized around Janie and her baby - meals are brought to her when it is convenient and desired; no one disturbs her sleep except her baby, she is in her own comfortable bed in her own room next to her own dear man. This is how birth was meant to be - custom-built for this woman. Here she is unique, the only one, not one of dozens trying to learn the 'ward routine'. Here she is the queen, the pivot, the most important person - the *mother.*

Reproduced with kind permission from Primary Health Care, April 1986

Retracing Our Cultural Roots

The culture of childbirth is being ignored, says Caroline Flint. She calls for a greater awareness of cultural differences in the experience of childbirth and argues that this need not impinge on the safety of the baby

We care about our culture. Each nation tries to preserve its cultural heritage. Go to Wales and you will see signs in the Welsh language and hear people speaking in Welsh. Go to Ireland and you will hear the Erse being spoken. Go to Scotland and you can hear Gaelic being spoken and a cultural heritage being preserved.

Our cultural heritage is important and we realize this and preserve it. It gives us a sense of our own history. It gives us a sense of identity. It is a necessary part of our culture. And yet, what seems to me to be the most important part of culture, the tap root of our society and how that society functions, is missing.

The way we are born and the way we give birth seem to have been neglected as part of our culture. While we have been carefully cherishing music, art, paintings, endangered species of animals and birds, ancient manuscripts and even old vacuum cleaners, the cultural heritage of how we give birth and how we are born has been totally ignored.

Not only do we alienate ourselves from our own cultural heritage when we apply no sensitivity to the way in which we give birth, but also many women who come into our hospitals to give birth come from a different cultural background from the indigenous population. All too often we give no respect to how each women would normally give birth, how she would normally move, what she would normally eat, who she would normally have with her, what she learned at her mother's knee.

Bardon[1] talks about giving birth as being genetically learned, in the way that a child can ride a bike easily because his mother and father learned to ride a bike. And in the same way that our great grandchildren will not even think about 'learning how to use computers'. It will be part of their genetic makeup. What are we doing to the genetic imprinting of birth?

Birth is very much part of our culture.

I recently watched some colourful Bulgarian dancing. With it, there was a photographic exhibition, which included a photo showing about 30 babies in cribs attended by women in nurses' uniforms. The caption underneath proudly stated, 'All mothers in Bulgaria are delivered in modern, well equipped clinics.' There babies, many of whom seemed to be crying miserably, were separated from their mothers. They were well fed, clean, and in modern cribs, but still separated from the source of their comfort.

I was reminded of an article about traditional birth attendants in India, which stated that the traditional birth attendants used dirty cloths for the labouring woman to sit on and used an unsterilized blade to cut the baby's cord. Having criticised these two unsavoury practices, the author concluded that all women should be delivered in hospital.

But does this necessarily mean that all births should automatically take place in hospital?

If all that is needed to ensure a safer delivery in the case of these particular traditional midwives is for them to wash the birth cloths and sterilise the blade, surely less upheaval would be caused by educating them in these two matters? This would seem to be preferable to uprooting the labouring woman and transferring her and her family – because when I was in India it appeared to me that most of the family went to hospital with the patient – to a hospital which could be miles away, and where she would be confronted with an American delivery bed complete with lithotomy poles. This is frightening enough for a western woman. But for the modest Indian woman, who may well be illiterate and speak in a different dialect to her caregivers, and who is used to squatting to eat, to wash clothes, to wash dishes, to cook, to chat, to prepare food – what a humiliation it must be for her to lie strapped down, with her genitalia exposed to the world!

The thought is unbearable. So many of the women told me horror stories about the hospitals, and yet many of the trained nurse/midwives told me horror stories about the traditional birth attendants. I was conscious of seeing a culture being destroyed, and I realized I was only seeing a repeat of what has happened here in Britain over the past 50 years, and indeed is still happening.

Here, very few women give birth in their homes. Very few children can say, as my son used to say as he ushered visitors into our house, 'This is the bed I was born on.' Nor, as my daughter once did with a new boyfriend, 'We'll go on a tour of the houses my brothers and I were born in and I'll point out the rooms we were born in.' Birth is very much a part of our culture. By alienating women from it, we are doing something which will affect our whole culture.

Some would say that we are doing it for the safety of the baby, but this is not necessarily true. As MacVicar said in 1981[2], more women having babies in this decade come into an obstetric low risk category than ever before in our history. We need to remember that those of us who interfere with something so basic to our roots as childbirth need to take care when we transplant the plant wholesale. Plants, like cultures, are delicate and need to be treated with respect.

References
1. Bardon, D. Speaking at the 25th birthday conference of the Association for Improvement in the Maternity Service. November 29, 1985.
2. MacVicar, J. (1981). 'Changing birth patterns during a period of declining births.' *Maternal and Child Health*; 6: 7, pp. 280-284.

Reproduced with kind permission from Nursing Times, March 18, 1987

The Case for Home Birth

Childbirth is very much a normal part of life. All of us were children and were born to mothers and fathers; many of us are mothers or fathers ourselves; it is an integral part of life and of the community. Babies are conceived in our own beds or on our own sitting room floors and pregnancy takes place during everyday life - there is a pregnant woman on the bus, the local shop assistant is pregnant, and the woman next door.

When the woman next door has her baby it will grow up next door, it will be breast or bottle-fed in the house next door, it will be loved and guided and sent to school and take exams and start work all from the house next door.

In 1987 the only event in that family's life together which will not happen in the house next door is the birth of that baby.

If this were obligatory for safety no-one would question the wisdom of putting a woman into an alienating environment for her confinement. Yet more and more evidence is challenging whether a hospital actually is the safest place for the normal low-risk woman to have her baby.

I have worked as a midwife in hospitals considered to be among the foremost in trying to humanize the environment. Nevertheless I have observed that the accumulation of expensive equipment in a maternity hospital makes it almost obligatory for it to be used, such as electronic fetal monitoring and ultrasound. Both have some benefits, especially for women at risk, but their validity for women going through an uncomplicated pregnancy and labour remains very much in question.

Hospital also means bed - when women are admitted in labour they are almost automatically put into a bed which is probably not a sensible position.

The effects of gravity on the fetus encourage the dilation of the cervix; and lying in bed means the uterus is leaning back on the great blood vessels of the body and so restricting the circulation to the fetus.

Imagine the difference when a woman is labouring at home. Instead of going somewhere strange, the woman is visited by the midwife. She will be watching television, sitting in the garden, in the bath, lying on her bed in whatever position she has chosen to adopt. It will be her choice, and the equipment to help her take up her chosen position is there in her own house - ordinary settees, baths, cushions, carpets or stools.

At home the woman is an individual. Because the environment is hers and the midwife is the guest, the relationship between them is subtly altered. When the midwife wants to do something to the woman she will automatically explain and ask her permission. Yet a woman who steps inside a maternity institution has to undergo a wide range of routine tasks as a matter of course, often without explanation.

Some of these routines are appropriate and right for some women, not for all. Many of them are inappropriate and unevaluated. Apart from the ethical questions, the implications of giving all women certain treatments are enormous.

Today when most homes have hot and cold running water and satisfactory heating and when most women are fit and healthy during pregnancy, it is sensible to compare the cost of keeping a woman in hospital with that of caring for her at home.

Staying in a hospital bed for 24 hours costs a minimum of £160. Most women are in labour for up to a day and, according to the Hospital In-patient Enquiry (Maternity) the average length of stay after delivery is 5.5 days. For the average woman the cost to the NHS is a minimum of £880, plus the cost of antenatal care, being in the delivery suite, fetal monitoring (£6 for scalp electrode, £4 for the recording paper) and analgesia. Add the cost of her partner's visits by bus, train or car and it can be seen that the decision to deliver all women in hospital was a very expensive one. In comparison, the cost of a community midwife at the top of her salary scale, with the additional costs of her car, phone and uniform, is no more than £60 a day.

Recent evidence supports a greater use of community midwives. Campbell has assessed every birth taking place at home in 1979. Not surprisingly, she found that those women who had not booked into hospital and who had not booked a community midwife were at very great risk, with a perinatal mortality rate (infant deaths) of 196.9 per 1,000.

Surprisingly, those who had booked for a hospital confinement and then delivered at home, either because of a precipitate labour or because they didn't leave for hospital in time, had a high perinatal mortality rate of 67.5 per 1,000.

But perhaps the greatest surprise to those who believe that babies can only be delivered safely in hospital was the perinatal mortality rate for those women who had booked with a community midwife and who had their babies at home - 4.1 per 1,000. Campbell surmises that if she had been able to find out what happened to the 10 per cent who were transferred to hospital, their perinatal mortality would probably have doubled to 8 per 1,000 - showing that a booked home confinement is a safe option for the woman at low risk of complications.

Damstra-Wijmenga looked at women who had opted for a home confinement in 1981 in Holland, comparing their results with a group of comparatively low risk women. The women who delivered at home experienced much less professional intervention than the comparable group in hospital, and their babies were born in better condition. He suggests that women at low risk may be in danger of hospital-induced complication when entering an institution which is geared to the pathology of birth.

Klein has shown how women and their babies have fared much better when assessed in early labour either at their home or in the GP's surgery by a community midwife. They actually had longer labours than women in a comparable group who had all their labour care in the obstetric unit, but they went into the maternity unit more advanced in labour; they received less analgesia; they had fewer instrumental deliveries; their babies had higher Apgar scores and less need of admission to special care.

Tew analysed the results of the most recent survey of British births (1970). She suggested that even when allowance is made for greater numbers of women at greater predelivery risk when looking at the figures for hospital births, perinatal mortality is significantly higher in consultant units than at home or in GP units. The outcry to refute her findings was speedy and shrill, but Tew is a statistician of standing and no-one has yet produced facts to disprove hers.

Women have been asked about where they would prefer to give birth, in recent surveys carried out by *Woman's Hour* and the Health Visitors Association. Fourteen per cent said they would prefer to give birth at home; and this is after 15 years of intensive conditioning on the part of the medical profession that birth should take place in hospital. Perhaps the time has come to review this philosophy.

If the selection of women for home birth is sensible, including only those who have good social support, are nutritionally sound, are over five feet tall, have had no uterine surgery and no medical complications, the results should be excellent as long as there are good facilities for easy transfer to hospital. Women could give birth in the comfort and peace of their own homes, the midwife could be happy in her role and the NHS could use the money saved.

If we are not yet ready for this step, perhaps it is worth looking at Klein's ideas for assessing women at home in early labour. As O'Driscoll says, 'the most important single item in the management of labour is diagnosis' perhaps by assessing women at home we should have fewer women in our labour wards who are not really in established labour. And how comforting it would be to a woman when she rings in the night wondering if she is really in labour to hear the reply 'All right, we'll send the midwife round'.

We should be looking at birth at home as a viable choice for women - some randomized controlled trials along the lines of the Know Your Midwife project at St George's Hospital in Tooting, London. A group of five or six midwives could work together and look after 200-250 women a year throughout pregnancy, labour and the puerperium. A list of criteria (as suggested above) should be drawn up and 750 women a year should be selected as suitable for home delivery; the women could be randomized on a 1:2 basis so that annually 250 women would be the control group having their babies in hospital, as at present, and 500 would be offered birth at home.

In the present climate half of these women would refuse, leaving three groups: 250 having babies in hospital, 250 having their babies at home and 250 who were offered a home-birth but opted for hospital. The results could be analysed over a four-year period giving a realistic evaluation of home birth. It is also of paramount importance to find out how the women feel about the experience and what their preferences are.

There are currently around 157,000 qualified midwives but only 26,500 are practising - one out of every five. This huge wastage represents a tragedy of lost hopes and lack of job satisfaction. If my suggestions could be practised, would we have room for all the midwives who would come rushing back, as well as enormous benefits to mothers and babies?

References

Caldeyro-Barcia. *Physiological and psychological bases for the modern and humanized management of normal labour.* Scientific Publication No. 858, Centro Latinoamericano de Perinatologia y Desarrollo Humano.

Campbell, R. (1984). 'Home births in England and Wales, 1979: perinatal mortality according to intended place of delivery', *British Medical Journal, 289,* 22 September.

Damstra-Wijmenga, S. (1984). 'Home confinement: the positive results in Holland', *Journal of the Royal College of General Practitioners,.*

Klein, M. (1983). 'A comparison of low-risk pregnant women booked for delivery in two systems of care: shared care (Consultant) and integrated general practice unit', *British Journal of Obstetrics and Gynaecology,* 90, pp.118-128.

Tew, M. (1985). 'Place of birth and perinatal mortality', *Journal of the Royal College of General Practitioners,* .

Flint, C. (1985). 'Labour of love', *Nursing Times,* January 30 and Poulengeris, P. (1985). 'Under the microscope', *Nursing Times,* February 6.

O'Driscoll, K.(1980). *Active Management of Labour,* W.B. Saunders.

Reproduced with kind permission from Socialism and Health, Spring 1987

Home Service

More and more women want to have their babies at home away from an institutional environment. But, says Caroline Flint, midwives are still pushing mothers into hospital confinements for no good reason

I was talking to three women who all live in the same district of London. They had all had a baby in the past few months – at home – with an independent midwife. Why hadn't any of them had a community midwife I asked. Mary looked angry. 'You have to be joking', she said. 'I asked for a home birth week after week, and every midwife I saw said that you couldn't have a baby at home if it was your first baby. Finally, I got through to the midwife in charge of the community midwives. She said that it was possible to have your first baby at home, but that you had to be checked by a consultant obstetrician. When I saw him he said that he didn't agree with first-time mothers having babies at home. I had so much hassle that in the end I decided to have my baby at home with just my husband and not to call anyone. Then I heard about Becky (an independent midwife) and rang her. We found it difficult to pay even though she brought her fees right down.'

Angie had been expecting her second baby and the reason that she had been refused a home birth was that she had had high blood pressure during her first pregnancy (not repeated at all during her second pregnancy except on the day she had waited for hours in the antenatal clinic). Claudia had been refused a home birth because she had had a forceps delivery during her first pregnancy.

I discussed these three women with the independent midwife. She told me that many women in her area were being strongly discouraged from having a baby at home. It was really too far away from her home for her to take on cases there, but she couldn't bear to refuse after the stories the women told her.

What made me so sad was that these women had approached members of my own profession, and instead of receiving support and guidance, they had been flung into a system resembling a type of Chinese torture. They were being told: 'To have a baby at home you must comply with this – and now this – and now this – and so on. On what evidence was this done?

Where to be born? The debate and the evidence, a report recently published by the National Perinatal Epidemiology Unit[1], looks at the results of delivering women in different places over the past century and comes up with several conclusions. Perhaps the most significant is that: 'There is no evidence to support the claim that the safest policy is for all women to give birth in hospital'. It also concludes that: 'The policy of closing down small obstetric units on the grounds of safety is not supported by the available evidence'.

It goes on to suggest that 'there is some evidence, although not conclusive, that morbidity is higher among mothers and babies cared for in an institutional setting. For some women, the iatrogenic risk associated with institutional delivery may be greater than any benefit conferred, but this has yet to be proven'.

As midwives we should remember our name, mid-wife – with woman. We should be by her side, supporting and strengthening her, and preparing her for the job of motherhood.

This is reflected in the latest publication from the Royal College of Midwives, *Towards a healthy nation – a policy for the maternity services*[2], which comes up with several refreshingly flexible models on which midwives could base their case of pregnant women. 'The college now recognizes the fact that there is some doubt about the assumption that the safest place for delivery of all women is invariably a consultant unit', it states.

It also recommends that 'a recognized home confinement service should exist in all health authorities, and that maternity units should provide a range of delivery facilities to meet the various needs of all women through the spectrum of low to high risk.'

Women and midwives are getting together. What women say is being heard at long last. But is everyone hearing it?

I have read recently about the Royal College of Gynaecologists' document on delivering women in this age of AIDS which suggests that the midwife should wear a visor, a plastic apron, full length gown, and boots (I had never realised that you could catch AIDS via your feet, or abdomen and thighs for that matter).[3]

I would have thought that a more relevant conclusion would be that we need to protect ourselves and the baby against needle-stick injuries. This means that we need to be thinking twice before artificially rupturing membranes, applying fetal scalp electrodes and performing fetal blood sampling. That is much more relevant than wearing a gown from head to foot.

References
1. Campbell, R. and Macfarlane, A. (1987). *Where to be born? The debate and the evidence.* National Perinatal Epidemiology Unit, Radcliffe Infirmary, Oxford.
2. The Royal College of Midwives. *Towards a healthy nation – a policy for the maternity services.* London: RCM.
3. Hodgkinson, N. (1987). 'AIDS alert in maternity wards.' *Sunday Times,* May 31.

Reproduced with kind permission from Nursing Times, June 17, Vol 83, No 24, 1987.

No Place like Home for Labour

Last summer I looked after a woman in labour (her first) and spent the greater part of her labour lounging in the sun on her roof garden. She was just a floor away when she needed me she could call. When I heard signs that she needed me, I immediately went to her aid and comfort. Every half an hour or so I checked the baby' heart. The labour progressed; the young mother and father massaged, comforted and strengthened each other during the long hours - private, self-contained, intimate.

Yesterday I was at another first labour. It was, like most other labours, fairly long and gruelling; the young couple supported each other, drawing on strengths that neither knew the other possessed. They spent hours alone together quietly in their room while my partner and I spent the hours in the sitting room, knitting, chatting quietly, sipping tea, reminiscing about other labours we had attended, discussing the forthcoming election, the state of midwifery, the state of the world. During the conversation I asked myself why we were a floor away from the labouring woman, able to hear her groaning, able to respond immediately if she called or cried out in distress, able to be at her side within seconds. Why weren't we at her side all through?

The reason that we weren't at her side all the time, and why I hadn't continuously been at the first woman's side, was that we had felt from each woman that she needed privacy and an opportunity to be alone with her beloved. We had left them to draw on their own resources. Of course we checked the baby's heart and we kept an eye on the mother

and her physical condition - was her bladder empty, was she coping with the contractions, was she relaxed and in a good position and good spirits? But coming through overwhelmingly was her need to be alone with the only person who would not be intruding on this intimate experience.

This led me to discuss the situation with my partner. She reminded me that when I looked after women in labour in hospital I never leave their sides. If I am hungry I eat my banana/sandwich/chocolate bar in the room with them; if I am thirsty I drink my tea/coffee/slimmasoup with them. I never leave their sides for a moment except for what my husband invariably calls 'physical needs relief' (an old busman's term). Why do I treat women at home so differently from those in hospital? Surely some of the women in hospital were in need of privacy just as at home.

The reason, I now realize, is because I am protecting women in hospital from interference.

Taking a break

If I should mosey off for a tea break, a coffee break or even a knitting session in front of the hospital television it is highly likely that someone may enter the bedroom that my couple are in

"You look as though you are in pain would you like an epidural/pethidine/entonox', the mother may be told, or even 'Why haven't you got a monitor on - let's put one on you - please get up on to the bed' or even 'You've been a long time, it would be a good idea to hurry things along'

127

So when I came back from my tea break I should find the woman, who had been perfectly all right and coping well with the contractions of labour, with an intravenous drip in situ, her membranes ruptured and well on the way to having an epidural. As for the active position she had wanted to take up and which had enabled her to cope with contractions - she is now lying on the bed, not to be able to get up again until after the birth of her baby. Her labour is being accelerated, her pain increased and more difficult to cope with and her need for strong analgesia is greater. Fine if that is what she wanted but often it is not and so often it happens if she is left unattended by her midwife.

Familiarity.
The other difficulty of leaving a couple on their own in a labour ward is that they do not know where you are. When I was sitting on Hannah's roof garden or yesterday in Judy's sitting room, the room is familiar to the woman. She can picture me there and she knows I am only a groan away.

She is aware if I am sitting on the settee or the lounger; she would be aware if I helped myself to a record to play or got a magazine out of the rack because women know what is going on in their house. That is why they always come leaping up the stairs when the toddler has gone quiet, even though they were not really aware that he was up there in the first place.

Privacy - some women need it badly during labour, others like to be massaged and stroked and cuddled. But once again I have been made aware of the huge differences when a woman has her baby at home compared to the hustle and bustle that she must endure at her hospital birth.

Perhaps there are some hospitals which have enabled women to have privacy in labour - is there any unit out there where the delivery rooms have a bolt for the doors? Is there anywhere in the United Kingdom where women can labour in private without people barging in, with the most benign of motives, to offer a cup of tea, to see if equipment is free.

Even so, each time a woman in labour is interrupted so is her labour. Labouring women need privacy, can they get it anywhere but at home ?

Reproduced with kind permission from Primary Health Care, June 1987

Birth Control?

The debate over hospital versus home birth is highlighted in a document from the National Epidemiology Unit. Caroline Flint examines the evidence in the report

A woman who wants to have her baby at home these days causes hackles to rise. She may be told, 'but I didn't think you were allowed to any more?', 'isn't that a bit foolhardy?', or 'isn't it illegal?' But this attitude hasn't always been the case.

A new report, *Where to Be Born*[1], shows that until the late 1960s, having a baby at home was a normal and frequent choice made by women and indeed a decision to go into a hospital to have a baby was attended by many hazards. Florence Nightingale wrote in 1871, 'With all their defects, midwifery statistics point to one truth; namely, that there is a large amount of preventable mortality in midwifery practice, and that, as a general rule the mortality is far, far greater in lying-in hospitals than among women lying-in at home.'

Such observations run through the report, countered by arguments that the high risk women congregate in hospital so that the increased mortality rate is to be expected.

The report documents the landslide to hospital birth which occurred as recently as the 1950s when the Ministry of Health said, 'While demands for hospital beds for acute cases, tuberculosis and other serious conditions cannot be met adequately in many areas, it is difficult to justify the provision of hospital accommodation for normal maternity cases simply because the mother prefers to have her baby in hospital.' At the end of the decade, 36 per cent of women were still having their babies at home.

The report cites a plethora of documents concerned with maternity, some of which advise home birth as safer than hospital birth. But scientific reasons are rarely given and, in fact, comparison of outcomes between home and hospital is actively discouraged in some of the reports. 'A direct comparison of the safety to mother and child in hospital delivery as opposed to domiciliary confinement, as at present organized, is vitiated because known difficult cases are normally booked for hospital and emergencies are rushed there. In fact, in any such comparisons, it is usual for the death rates to be higher in hospital than at home, though no informed person would adduce this particular fact as evidence that it is more dangerous to have a baby in hospital. On the contrary, in the present circumstances, there would be general agreement that, from a medical point of view, obstetrical cases which are likely to have material complications should deliver in hospital.' (1956)

The report is critical of other studies which base their recommendations on questionable information – for example, when 'place of booking' is assessed rather than 'place of delivery'. Obviously when a woman booked for a home birth has complications, she is transferred to hospital. The outcome of this patient needs to be assessed differently to those women who book for hospital and who have their baby there.

The report looks at evidence from GP units that other reports have used. The perinatal mortality in these units is extremely low, but it is presumed this has more to do with 'good selection' of women than the quality of care received.

The conclusions of the report are blunt. 'There is no evidence to support the claim that the safest policy is for all women to give birth in hospital ...' There is some evidence, although this is not conclusive, that morbidity is higher among mothers and babies cared for in an institutional setting. For some women, the iatrogenic risk associated with institutional delivery may be greater than any benefit conferred, but this has yet to be proven.'

How timely is the other new report from the Royal College of Midwives, *Towards a Healthy Nation – a policy for the maternity services*[2]. It says that hospital provision for all deliveries is 'not a realistic objective' and 'it is appropriate for maternity service planning to allow for a proportion of low-risk women to be delivered at home. The implication of this is that home confinements should not be undertaken on an *ad hoc* basis but that a recognized home confinement service should exist in all health authorities'.

These proposals are similar to those made by the Association of Radical Midwives which published a report in 1986, *The Vision – proposals for the future of the maternity services*[3] which said that, 'Midwives in group practices would deliver women in hospital and at home, according to individual circumstances and individual choice.'

Women, midwives, GPs and obstetricians will be grateful to Rona Campbell and Alison Macfarlane for this comprehensive and scientific look at what happens to women having babies in this country and perhaps the report points out the need for further investigation into policies for pregnant women in the UK based on reason and scientific research.

References
1. Campbell, R., Macfarlane, A. (1987) *Where To Be Born. The debate and the evidence.* National Perinatal Epidemiology Unit, Radcliffe Infirmary, Oxford.
2. The Royal College of Midwives.(1987) *Towards a Healthy Nation – a Policy for the Maternity Services.* London: RCM, .
3. Association of Radical Midwives.(1986). *The Vision – Proposals for the Future of the Maternity Services.* Ormskirk, ARM.

Reproduced with kind permission from Nursing Times, July 15, Vol 83, No 28, 1987

Delivery at Home

Allowing women who wish to have a home delivery may make them feel more relaxed and secure during labour, says Caroline Flint

On the day you read this article, 20 babies will be born at home in England and Wales. This is a small number with the 1,580 who will be born in hospital. But it is likely that each birth at home represents a struggle by the parents to achieve having their baby at home.

They may have had the senior midwife coming to their house to 'test' their commitment to home birth by trying to persuade them to have their baby in hospital and leave soon after the birth. They may have had an emotional reaction from their GP who probably doesn't favour birth at home. The midwife who attends them may have spent time initially trying to persuade them to have the baby in hospital. On the other hand, she may have arranged for them to see a GP who was not their usual one so that they had a sympathetic GP to support them.

They may, to their surprise, have had their request treated as normal. The midwife may have been pleased at their decision. Or they may have engaged an independent midwife who does nothing else but home births. Or their GP may be one of the few in this country who favours birth at home and supports women asking for it.

Brave

Whichever way, the decision will have caused a stir among the couple's friends and relatives. They will have been besieged by people telling them how brave they are.

Home birth is such an emotive subject that it never goes unremarked. Despite the numerically few births at home in 1989, their effect is all out of proportion to their numbers.

Why? What is it about birth at home that is so controversial? Why do people choose to have their baby at home?

I sometimes reminisce on my choice of a home birth for my first child in 1965. Having worked in maternity hospitals, I knew that they were not restful places and that women had problems in sleeping when so many mothers and babies were crammed into one large room.

So the main reason for my choice of a home birth was that I wanted as much rest as possible after the birth – to sleep in my own bed with my own dear man beside me.

Shared event

That also is a great benefit of having a baby at home – both parents learn together how to bath a baby, how to change its nappy, the delights of winding. The father of the baby also has a greater part to play in providing care for his wife: cooking her meals, washing sheets, knickers, endless babygrows. It may be exhausting, but it makes the birth of the baby, and the becoming of a family, a shared event right from the start.

In 1965, I had no problem in arranging for a home birth, since about 30 per cent of women had their babies at home in those days. It was an accepted part of life. No-one suggested that I was brave or even foolhardy; I was just having a baby.

Another reason for choosing a home birth is to stay in control of the situation. Even in labour, the woman is the hostess. The medical personnel are the visitors.

It is the mother's house, her domain. Even what is available to drink and the availability of clean towels is controlled by her. For some women, this is a paramount reason for a home birth. They don't want anything 'done to them' without their willing agreement, and it is extremely hard for this to happen to them in their own home.

Safer

A more recent reason for choosing to have a home birth is that some women genuinely feel their baby will be safer at home than in hospital. Some women become frightened by the number of 'routine' procedures which are likely to come their way if they give birth in hospital. They feel they may be putting their baby at risk.

An instance is the routine rupture of membranes at a certain stage of cervical dilation, which is common in many hospitals. Many women are well versed in the literature surrounding childbirth and aware of the work of Kitzinger and Caldeyro Barcia.

They have shown that artificial rupturing of membranes increases pain of labour, decreases the women's ability to cope with the pain of labour and is more likely to end in an instrumental delivery than when the membranes are left intact to rupture spontaneously (usually at the end of the first stage of labour).

Women know about the work of Kumar and Robson which shows that when women have their membranes ruptured artificially during labour they are less likely to feel attachment to their baby and more likely to feel distant from their baby. Women want their baby to be born in optimal conditions and they don't trust that these are necessarily the conditions which prevail in their local maternity unit.

This sentiment was voiced in the controversial gathering together of research and studies into birth made by Campbell and McFarlane. They propose that, according to all the available data: 'There is no evidence to support the claim that the safest policy is for all women to give birth in hospital'.

Morbidity

An equally compelling statement is that 'There is some evidence though not conclusive, that morbidity is higher among mothers and babies cared for in an institutional setting'.

Even with the large body of research which has now been amassed to show that childbirth at home is a safe option, many people are frightened by the prevailing philosophy in maternity care – 'What if something goes wrong?'

The whole of maternity care at this moment is geared to this concept of abnormality and pathology. Surely, with those thoughts uppermost in the care-givers minds, it is *more* likely that things go wrong.

Women are so susceptible during pregnancy and labour, it is surely much easier to be at home with the concept that 'things will go well'. Then, if things do begin to go badly, transfer to hospital is in order.

References
Schwarcz, R. and Caledyro-Barcia, R. (1887). 'Amniotomy', in Anderson, Chalmers and Turnbull (Eds). *Elective Delivery in Obstetric Practice,* Oxford University Press.
Campbell, R. and MacFarlane, A.(1987). *Where To Be Born: The Debate and the Evidence,* Oxford: National Perinatal Epidemiology Unit.

Further Reading
Robson, K.M. (1982). 'I feel nothing' *Nursing Mirror,* June 23.

Reproduced with kind permission from Nursing, October 12–25, Vol. 3, No. 43, 1989

Labour

The importance for a woman to be in control of her own childbearing

For most women becoming a mother is the most important and most powerful role that she will ever take on. To a small child his mother is like a goddess – she is the source of all knowledge, the source of all nourishment, the source of all power, the source of all self esteem. To the small child and infant, the mother is a marvellous, exciting, amazing person, the source of delight and love.

To take on this very powerful and demanding role it is obvious that a woman needs to be brimming over with self confidence, she needs to feel strong both physically and emotionally, she needs to feel in control of the situation.

When examined closely, the way in which we provide care for pregnant women at the present time actually puts the woman at an enormous disadvantage when taking on the role of being a mother. It is almost as if we had designed a regime which makes women feel powerless and overwhelmed – at a time when they need to feel more powerful than at any time in their lives.

Maternity care is provided to woman in alien surroundings, at times which are convenient to us, and often inconvenient for them, in hospitals which for most people represent illness, pain and death. At every stage of this tender sequence we surround her with strangers.

When labour starts the woman leaves the warmth and familiarity of her home, her own place which smells of her, feels like hers and is hers and she travels to the hospital, to be greeted by a midwife she has never met before, who ushers her into a room – the like of which she has no experience.

Human beings are mammals – mammals need a sanctuary to labour and give birth in. They need somewhere dark and private with only their most intimate friend or relatives with them. The last place a mammal would choose to labour is in transit between home and hospital and then on what amounts to a high platform, under bright lights, observed by many, with people interrupting the process frequently by entering the room to enquire over progress, need for analgesia, need for refreshment, need for the midwife to answer the telephone.

Perhaps it is time for us to look again at what we now regard as the normal way of having a baby, and think about how it would or could be for the women if they were in a powerful position during their pregnancy and labour.

The woman is totally in control of the situation when she employs her own independent midwife to deliver her in her own home – and when examining this model several factors come up in that pattern of care which are worth thinking through.

When a woman engages an independent midwife the midwife comes to the woman's home, on the first visit it is to be 'looked over'. The woman may not take to her and may not engage her. All this is the woman's decisions, she is the employer and the midwife is a visitor in her house. The relationship starts from this basis – that the woman is the hostess and the employer, she is in charge.

The midwife will practice her profession to the best of her ability and will advise as necessary, but the bottom line is that the woman can either take or reject that advice – the midwife must continue with her care (United Kingdom Central Council for Nursing, Midwifery and Health Visiting, 1986), at the same time informing the Supervisor of Midwifery. At all times it is the woman's decision which counts – the woman holds the position of power.

Antenatal consultations will normally be held in the woman's home at a time which is convenient for her and her partner. She may be seen in the evening when her partner is available or during the day or at the weekend. She will have notes which are seen as a diary of pregnancy, labour and puerperium to be written in by the midwife, the man and the woman – there will be space specifically for the couple to chronicle the progress of their pregnancy. At the end of the postnatal visits at 28 days the woman will be given a photocopy of her notes to keep as a record of this pregnancy and labour.

When the woman is in control of her labour she telephones the midwife when she thinks she is in labour, they arrange when the midwife will come to the house. During the labour the woman takes up whatever position she wants and most women are extremely active, roaming around the house or the flat, often rocking and rotating their pelvis quite instinctively and thus changing and enlarging the pelvic diameters (Dunn, 1976; Russell, 1982). The woman is surrounded by furniture which she has brought specifically for her comfort, bean bags or a leather sofa or plain wooden chairs – the variety of homes is only equalled by the number of people who live in them – the place of labour is a place which she has designed for herself and her partner's needs –it is totally unique, there is no other place the same.

Equally, what the woman chooses to eat and drink during labour will be unique, she will have the sort of foods she likes and it can vary between crackle and pop cereal, to fruit spreads on bread, to macaroni pie, to soups, fruit teas, honey or tea and a biscuit. She is in charge of what she eats – she is in control of this aspect of her labour as she is with all other aspects of her labour.

The other factor of labouring in her own home surrounded by people she knows and trusts is that she can feel completely uninhibited either when she wants to make a noise or if she wants to remove her clothes, she can be in the bath, leaning against the worktop in the kitchen, or sitting on a sofa in front of the television having a cigarette (no place here for 'allowing' or not 'allowing') and watching the racing – it is her choice, she is in charge.

Our home is a place of sanctuary, total privacy is assured, no one comes in without an invitation, anyone who might disturb the peacefulness or the atmosphere of the labour is excluded.

After the delivery other factors increase the woman's self confidence. A few hours after the delivery the midwife leaves, she will have the instructed the woman and her partner into the intricacies of nappy changing and the baby will have suckled at the breast shortly after the delivery, but as she leaves the baby is left in the care of its parents and *they manage* . Many women stay awake following the birth gazing at their new baby, listening to every respiration, aware of every grunt and squeak, when the baby appears hungry the woman puts it to the breast and *she manages.*

From the very start the woman is this baby's mother and she learns to care for him or her. The woman learns that she has strong maternal instincts, learns that this baby is unique and she needs to learn how this baby ticks in the same way the baby is learning how to suck at these breasts, all this helps to increase the woman's perception of her own power and abilities.

If our concept of normality stemmed from this model – a woman in control of her own pregnancy consultations, labour and postnatal period, eating and drinking those foods she finds palatable, wearing or not wearing what she likes, surrounded by comfortable and familiar furniture – but above all assured of total privacy and attended by a midwife she has been able to get to know well for whom she is the employer, I suggest that our care even in hospital would change dramatically, and that it might keep pace with women's demands – they after all are the people who pay our salaries, who keep the National Health Service afloat with their taxes and who ultimately are our employer.

The time has come to encourage more women to have their babies at home – with a baseline of powerful women giving birth in their own surroundings – all those involved in childbirth would have a new baseline, a baseline of true 'normality' on which to base their care. The time has come – as is reflected on the following quotations;

'A recognized home confinement service should exist in all health authorities.' (Royal College of Midwives, 1987).

'Forms of care which should be abandoned in the light of the available evidence - Insisting on universal institutional confinement'. (Enkin et al., 1989).

'The recent results of maternity care in Holland reliably confirm what might have been surmised from the earlier results there – that midwives, practising their skills in human relations and without sophisticated technological aids, are the most effective guardians of childbirth and that the emotional security of a familiar setting, the home, makes a greater contribution to safety than does the equipment in hospital to facilitate obstetric interventions in cases of emergency.' (Tew, 1989).

'Mothers are also nowadays almost always offered the option to give birth at home so long as there is sound medical advice to support that in each case.' (Clarke, 1989).

'Mrs Virginia Bottomly Health Minster opened the Conference – her message to the midwives was that their human and psychological skills must be used, and that women must have choice between giving birth at home, in a GP unit or in a hospital. (Bottomley, 1990.)

'It has never been scientifically proved that the hospital is a safer place than the home for a woman who has an uncomplicated pregnancy to have her baby. Studies of planned home births in developed countries with women who have had uncomplicated pregnancies have shown sickness and death rates for mother and baby equal or better than hospital birth statistics for women with uncomplicated pregnancies.' (World Health Organization,1985).

'The main findings in this survey of all births occurring at home in England and Wales in 1979 were the low perinatal mortality among births booked to occur at home and the considerably higher mortality among births booked for hospital or not booked at all.' (Campbell et al., 1984).

'It was shown that among women who had opted for home confinement significantly fewer complications occurred during pregnancy, delivery and puerperium than among those who had their babies in hospital followed by a 24-hour stay there or followed by a seven-day stay in a maternity ward. Morbidity was also lower among the babies born at home than among those born in hospital.' (Damstra-Wijmenga,1984).

There is no evidence to support the claim that the safest policy is for all women to give birth in hospital. There is some evidence, although not conclusive, that morbidity is higher among mothers and babies cared in for in institutional setting. For some women, the iatrogenic risk associated with institutional delivery may be greater than any benefit conferred, but this has yet to be proven. (Campbell and Macfarlane, 1987).

Only midwives know about birth at home, only midwives (except for a tiny tiny number of general practitioners) deliver babies at home, it is up to us to inform women of their right to have a baby at home – our name means 'with woman', it is time we let women know that undoubtedly there are risks in childbirth, but that the risks of a home birth are no greater than a hospital birth and for some women they are indeed less.

References

Bottomley, V. (1990). Minister of Health opening the Royal College of Midwives Annual Conference, July 1990. *Midwife, Health Visitor and Community Nurse,* November.

Campbell, R., Davies, J.M., MacFarlene, A., Beral, V. (1984) 'Home births in England and Wales, 1979: perinatal mortality according to intended place of delivery.' *British Medical Journal,* 289, pp. 721-724.

Campbell, R., MacFarlene, A. (1987). *Where to be born, The Debate and the Evidence.* Oxford, National Perinatal Epidemiology Unit.

Clarke, K., Secretary of State for Health. (1989). *The Guardian,* 21st September.

Damstra-Wijenga, S.M.I. (1984). 'Home confinement: the positive results in Holland.' *Journal of the Royal College of General Practitioners.* 34, pp.425-430.

Dunn, P.M (1976). 'Obstetric delivery today. For better or worse?' *Lancet i* pp.790-793.

Enkin, M., Keirse, M., Chalmers, I. (1989). *A Guide to Effective Care in Pregnancy and Childbirth.* Oxford: Oxford University Press.

Royal College of Midwives (1987). *Towards a Healthy Nation. A Policy for Maternity Services.* London.

Russell, J.G.B. (1982). 'The rationale of primitive delivery positions.' *British Journal of Obstetrics and Gynaecology,* 89, pp.712-715.

Tew, M. (1990). *Safer Childbirth?* London: Chapman and Hall.

United Kingdom Central Council for Nursing, Midwifery and Health Visiting, (1986). *A Midwife's Code of Practice* . London: UKCC.

World Health Organization (1985). *Having a Baby in Europe.* Geneva:WHO.

Reproduced with kind permission from Journal of Obstetrics and Gynaecology, March 1991.

Home Births for All

Caroline Flint suggests every woman should book for a home birth, whether she wants one or not

During every NCT class I take, I suggest to the assembled group, almost every week, that they should book for a home birth. Sometimes the class members get fed up with me wittering on about home births and they firmly tell me to shut up. Sometimes one or two people in the class change to a home birth. Sometimes I feel embarrassed about pushing home births so strongly because my daytime job (and night-time as well quite often) is that of an independent midwife, which means that I am midwife in private practice mainly delivering babies at home. So I am always aware that people might feel that I am promoting my own service, but because I feel so strongly about the advantages of home birth I ignore the implications that might be coming up and just press on recommending home births just the same.

When a woman books into a hospital it is presumed by that institution that she has taken on all the philosophies, all the policies, all the procedures that come with that hospital. The woman going into hospital saying 'I am planning on having a totally normal birth with no intervention at all' could actually be kidding herself if she is walking through the doors of a hospital which specializes in epidurals and the medicalization of birth. However pro-choice the hospital may try to be, in a big institution the needs of the institution always seem to take precedence over the needs of the individual.

So why do I suggest to everybody that they should book for a home birth? Am I just misleading them or could it have been a useful thing to have done? My contention is that, even if a woman wants to have her baby in hospital, even if she is planning to have an epidural, even if she ends up in hospital having a Caesarean section or a forceps or a ventouse delivery, it is always better to have booked at home.

If a woman books for a home birth she has everything set up and organized for having her baby at home. She has the number of the midwives that she can contact at any time of the day or night; she has the equipment in the home in case labour is very quick and the baby pops out at home; she has geared her whole house and family to having a baby and being in labour. On the day of the labour the woman can roam around the house leaning against different furniture, grumbling to herself and getting into comfortable positions in the certain knowledge that one of the midwives knows she is in labour and will be on her way.

Once the midwife arrives and assesses how the woman is progressing in labour, the labouring woman can decide where she is actually going to give birth. But because she is booked for a home birth if she decides to go into hospital for an epidural or because she needs an assisted delivery the midwife will expect to come with her. When she gets into hospital she will be branded as 'the woman who wanted a home birth', and everybody will then bend over backwards to make sure that the women's delivery is as pleasant and as comfortable and as unique as it would have been had she been able to stay at home.

If she then decides to leave the hospital three hours after delivery, although it is 2 o'clock in the morning – no-one will throw up their hands in horror, instead they will just presume that she is doing a perfectly normal and sensible thing because she was booked for a home birth anyway, and the staff would expect her to want to go home immediately.

By booking a home birth, even if a woman intends to have her baby in hospital, she has actually transcended the argument, discussion and difficulties many women face. Although it may be dishonest to book for a home birth when you are actually planning to have your baby in hospital, it does mean that you have some control over the situation.

One day the system will allow all women to have a named midwife who will be their ally and who will support them through the system. Until that time we need to use tactics to get around the system. I hope these suggestions will help.

Reproduced with kind permission from New Generation, September 1992.

Special Delivery Midwifery Practice

Caroline Flint describes the new independent midwife practice that she has set up with fellow midwife Valerie Taylor

We believe that women will not gain control over their births until more women give birth at home. At the moment there really is no choice of birth at home for the majority of women. The one per cent of women in the UK who end up having their baby at home are frequently unusually assertive and determined women who have sought out a midwife and /or doctor for their home birth and have delivered at home following a pregnancy during which many battles have been waged. Apart from these determined women, there are occasional pockets of continuing home births where either the GP or the local midwives have gone on delivering babies at home over the years and women really do have a valid choice.

The reasons for setting up Special Delivery Midwifery Practice are to make home births more 'mainstream', to increase the profile of birth at home, to make it something to which well motivated middle class women aspire, so that eventually it becomes something that all women consider.

By practising the midwife's role to the full the midwives also want to try to provide a role model of excellent midwifery practice – to this end they are committed to writing about and publishing the way in which they work, thus giving midwives a view of the full role of the midwife. Our personal aims also include earning a good living in a satisfying way.

Just another independent practice?

How does Special Delivery Midwifery Practice differ from any other independent midwifery practice? Could it be the same, only noisier? We are providing an independent service which offers: antenatal care (in the woman's home or office, or in Special Delivery's consulting rooms;) antenatal get-together groups; delivery pack; inco pads for floor and bed; blood tests; ultrasound scan; labour and delivery care by a known midwife; postnatal care for 28 days; photocopy of notes.

This is little different from other independent midwives' practice – one difference is that the blood tests and ultrasound scan are all done privately so that the midwives do not rely at all on the services of the NHS. Another difference is the provision of a Mother's Help for two weeks following the birth, for women delivering in London, (where the practice is based). The charge we make for the service is £1,950. For women who do not require a mother's help, the cost is £1,600 and for those living outside London, the cost is £1,450.

A national profile

Special Delivery Midwifery Practice has advertised nationally in order to let women know about the service. Every day women from all over the UK telephone asking for further information. These women are sent an Information Pack which comprises an introduction to the concept of having a baby at home. It gives Special Delivery Midwifery

Practice's own statistics – based on our previous independent practice and advises women to find out the statistics of wherever they decide to give birth or whoever they decide to have as their midwife or obstetrician.

In order to provide a service to women all over the country, we are compiling a list of midwives who are interested in carrying out the occasional home birth. Special Delivery Midwifery Practice has purchased several sets of up-to-date equipment for these midwives. They will introduce a midwife to interested women and will supply all equipment. This includes notes, blood tests and sample letters to GPs and supervisors of midwifery. As the aim is to increase the number and availability of home births, we feel that every time a midwife attends a home birth she sees birth for what it is, and gains a concept of the politics surrounding birth.

The expectant parents pay Special Delivery Midwifery practice for arranging this service and Special Delivery Midwifery Practice pay the midwife on the return of their equipment – thus enabling midwives to do the occasional independent birth with the support of two experienced home birth midwives, and without having the expense of buying all the equipment.

Most of the women contacting Special Delivery Midwifery Practice could not afford to pay for a private midwife – they are shown how to go about getting a home birth under the National Health Service and they are referred to the Society to Support Home Confinements or AIMS. Women going through this process feel able to telephone Special Delivery Midwifery Practice for further advice and ammunition in their quest for a birth at home. Their midwives are also encouraged to ring and discuss such topics as delivering a baby in water or when the woman is standing up.

One of the most popular aspects of the service is an initial consultation visit costing £50.00 with no obligation on either party. The initial consultation consists of one hour of the midwives' time, ideally face to face, but if necessary – over the phone. During this time the couple can explore every possibility to which they are entitled, both within and outside the NHS. They can receive unbiased opinion and advice on birth inside and outside hospital, and on different types of classes and preparation. If the couple go on to book Special Delivery Midwifery Practice the fee is deducted from the final total.

The service is more expensive than other independent midwifery services. The promotional literature and advertising costs have been greater than the costs incurred by most independent midwives, likewise the purchase of equipment. The legal costs of setting up a partnership and the cost of an accountant have been included, and during the writing up of the business plan the true costs of providing such a service have been calculated.

Hopefully everyone will benefit from this service. Home birth should achieve a higher profile, so that more women will be able to have one both inside and outside the NHS. Independent midwives should find more women coming to them to book, midwives wanting to 'test the water' will be able to carry out an independent home birth without the expense and anxiety usually associated with such a move. And hopefully, we will earn our living and increase our service until eventually we have several midwives working in Special Delivery Midwifery Practice. We will then be able to set up Birth Centres and ultimately, a Special Delivery Midwifery Training School.

Reproduced with kind permission from MIDIRS, March 1991.

Teams and Caseloads

Continuity of care has been the ruling passion of Caroline's professional life and this section bears witness to her ceaseless promotion of the concept over a period of fifteen years. The earliest article was written in 1979, shortly after Caroline had qualified as a midwife (having interrupted her training for 12 years whilst bearing and caring for her three children). She had immediately gone to work as a community midwife and had promised herself that she would work to change the face of maternity care within a decade.

These articles trace Caroline's thinking regarding continuity of care as it developed over the years. In 1979 she outlined a hospital-based scheme in which three midwives would provide care for 468 women per year throughout the antenatal and intranatal periods! ('A continuing labour of love'). This scheme was based on antenatal consultations lasting fifteen minutes and labour care averaging eight hours; unsurprisingly both calculations were revised thereafter. The scheme is presented in intricate detail, as are those which followed, and it is obvious that many, many hours of Caroline's life have been spent laboriously working out off-duty and holiday rosters and on-call and antenatal clinic schedules, with the idea that ready-devised packages were more likely to appeal to the sceptics amongst her professional colleagues.

The fact that *Nursing Mirror* made 'A continuing labour of love' its cover article nonetheless suggests that continuity of care was an idea likely to touch a chord with many midwives. In late 1981, shortly after getting the job of antenatal clinic sister at St George's Hospital in Tooting, Caroline wrote a series of four articles for *Nursing Mirror* in which she suggested a variety of ways in which continuity of care could be realized. Though still hospital-based, these schemes did carry continuity through the postnatal stay in hospital, and a more realistic woman to midwife ratio of 50-60: 1 per year. In addition to citing an improved experience of care for women, Caroline now also proposed that continuity of care would provide midwives with greater job satisfaction and also prove beneficial in financial terms, as well as possibly in terms of perinatal outcome.

At that time Caroline still saw her scheme as forming only a small service alongside conventional care within a maternity unit 'because it is too complicated and because high-risk patients need more care by doctors' ('Emma, Joan, Liz and A.N. Other'), a view she was to abandon by the time she helped reorganize care in Westminster and Kensington seven years later ('Riverside Midwife Teams'). She even gave half-hearted approval to the idea of teams of 15-16 hospital-based midwives formed around a consultant ('Small is intimate'), a model of care that was to give her the screaming ab-dabs by 1987 ('In search of continuity of care').

Meanwhile Caroline had taken on the job of antenatal clinic sister at a large London teaching hospital. Whilst still waiting to persuade someone to let her pilot a continuity of care scheme and to give her the necessary financial backing, she set about trying to improve conventional antenatal care and to introduce more continuity into the system. A series of nine articles describing her many and various ideas appeared in *Nursing Mirror* during the winter of 1982/ 83 ('Where have we gone wrong?'...'Encouraging feedback').

Public disgruntlement at maternity care has been picked up and projected by the media, and several thousand people had even gathered to demonstrate against one consultant's policies outside the Royal Free Hospital earlier in 1982. The fact that many of the ideas that Caroline put forward – taking histories in women's homes, birth-plans, midwives' clinics – were 'radical' goes to show the extent to which public disquiet was justified. The introduction of even a modicum of continuity into women's maternity care was not going to be easy.

In 1983, the effort Caroline had expended in developing a research proposal and applying for permission and funds to carry out a randomized controlled trial investigating continuity of care from a team of four midwives paid off. South West Thames Regional Health Authority and the Wellington Foundation awarded her the largest research grant ever made to a midwife in the UK. A number of articles outline and report on this original 'Know Your Midwife' (KYM) scheme, as it was named. Four midwives (though six midwives were actually involved over the two years of the trial) successfully gave care to 250 women a year from 1983-1985.

The KYM scheme was a watershed in midwifery and in Caroline's own life. It achieved what it set out to do in terms of the parameters of the study but all had not been plain-sailing. The report which appeared in *Nursing Times* in 1985 titled 'Labour of love' bears witness to some of the problems encountered by Caroline and her colleagues. Amongst these were disagreements with midwifery managers over the visiting of clients at home in early labour. This was eventually forbidden much to Caroline's despair. Another source of despondency was the suspension from practice of one of the team midwives over the unavoidable death of a baby. Somehow *Nursing Times* was persuaded to erase this midwife form the cover photograph on the edition in which 'Labour of love' appeared, leaving Caroline in tears of frustration, sadness and anger.

Furthermore, despite the positive findings of the KYM report, very few continuity of care schemes were developed in the years immediately following. In 1987, Caroline was publicly lamenting this fact ('How the midwife's role needs to change'). She herself, somewhat at a loose-end professionally, had gone into independent practice and undertaken the Advanced Diploma of Midwifery once the project had been completed. She was also, at this time, describing herself in the bits of biographical blurb accompanying her various articles as an independent midwife 'looking for a post in the Health Service where she can set up teams of midwives so that all women will know their midwives throughout the pregnancy and the postnatal period'. Riverside Health Authority took her on as a midwifery consultant shortly afterwards and with her help established what is probably, at the time of writing, the most fully developed system of team midwifery within the National Health Service.

In 1991 Caroline was appointed as one of two midwife advisors to the House of Commons Health Committee meeting under the chairmanship of Nicholas Winterton M.P to investigate the maternity services. The Winterton Committee's report of 1992 and, to a lesser extent, that of The Expert Maternity Group in 1993 represent the apotheosis of much of Caroline's long-held vision for maternity care. Nonetheless, her own thinking continues to develop and, by the time of the most recent article in the section ('Hailing a new philosophy'), she had come to see continuity in terms of midwifery caseloads whereby each midwife would care for 35 or 36 women a year and work in a partnership with one other midwife with a similar caseload.

During the years she spent at home caring for her children, Caroline had been a regular contributor to her parish magazine. It meant that by the time she relaunched herself into midwifery, she had developed the skill and zest for the written word which have been so essential to her vowed aim of radically changing midwifery. Her original time-scale of ten years may have been too optimistic but Caroline has made a vital impact on the profession she is so passionate about, and her willingness to put pen to paper (or fingers to keyboard) has been crucial in this. In no area is this more apparent than in continuity of care.

A Continuing Labour of Love

Caroline Flint describes her pilot for a scheme where three midwives co-operate in providing continuity of care for their patients - who would benefit from knowing the midwives who gave antenatal care and deliver the baby. The scheme would also improve the midwives' job satisfaction

Continuity of care is something we pay lip service to as being 'a good thing', something our patients desire very much[1], something only community midwives can achieve nowadays - but I believe continuity of care is far more important than we have so far realized.

With the use of ever more sophisticated monitoring of both the pregnant and the labouring woman in an attempt to lower the perinatal mortality rate, I think we may have lost sight of the most simple fact of all - that the same hand on the same abdomen every month (and then every week) picks up discrepancies which the usual medley of people who examine a pregnant woman easily miss.

We know the perinatal mortality rate rises with women who default from antenatal clinic attendance. One of the bonuses of continuity of care is that very few women miss an appointment; in my experience, if a woman does miss an appointment, she will turn up the following day or in a couple of days.

Why don't women miss antenatal visits when they are seeing a continuous person? Why do women want continuity of care? When they have it, why do they love it so?

My proposition is that in this situation the continuous person (that is, the midwife) can get to know each woman as an individual. When the patient comes into the room, she can be addressed by name, her worries or joys of the previous visit can be remembered. 'Hello, Joan, how did your move go?' or: 'Hello, Rachel, did your boyfriend get the job?' is a very different approach from: 'In here please, mother, and onto the scales.' Women appreciate being treated as individuals and respond with regular attendance.

Relaxed and realistic

Women experiencing continuity of care are more relaxed, they know their medical attendants as friends, they are not embarrassed or reticent in bringing up personal fears or worries, they feel more confident, and their expectations for labour can be discussed and noted - with realistic prospects that these can be carried out at the time.

I believe continuity of care could be the most decisive factor in the future reduction of the perinatal mortality rate, and probably the most influential factor in enhancing the quality of the experience of giving birth for both the expectant parents and their child.

How can we achieve continuity of care in the hospital setting? Can it be done? I believe it can - but that it needs a radical rethink in our use of midwife hours, and that it needs very special midwives to start the scheme. I also think that initially, and perhaps subsequently, not all patients could be included in it.

Involvement

Here is my plan for a pilot scheme achieving continuity of care throughout the antenatal period and during labour and delivery, by a team of three midwives. Between them, they can give antenatal care to and deliver 468 patients a year, and following delivery they can visit their patients in the postnatal wards.

The midwives will be working flexitime, coming in to their patients when they are needed but having definite off-duty days and on-call days so that they can plan their lives in advance.

This pilot scheme is for continuity of care during the antenatal period and delivery, but obviously the ideal would be to carry the concept through into postnatal care too. I would welcome suggestions and comments on how this could be achieved.

Emma becomes the first continuity midwife. She has been employed specifically to inaugurate the scheme and thus she needs to be someone who is settled in her private life (she will need to be involved in the scheme for at least two years to see any results), she needs to be on the telephone and she needs a car for which she is paid at the standard user rate.

Emma will be employed for 40 hours a week or 80 hours a fortnight. She will control her own off-duty and may find it helpful to have a clock-on, clock-off card or a card she fills in with the times she comes on or goes off duty.

Let us imagine that Emma starts working in the antenatal clinic in March. In the first month, she books 36 patients who are 12 weeks pregnant (nine a week) and explains to them about the continuity scheme. The continuity patients are allotted 15 minutes for every antenatal visit and Emma does all their care except that on their visits at 16 weeks, 32 weeks and at term, the patients also see the consultant obstetrician. Emma takes histories, weighs the patients, tests urine, takes blood pressures, tests for oedema and palpates the women's abdomens.

The following month (April), the 36 patients return and Emma also books another 36 patients who are 12 weeks pregnant. In May, Emma antenatals the 36 20-week pregnant patients, the 36 16-week pregnant

patients and books 36 12-week pregnant patients and so on.

Patients seen in June
  36 at 24 weeks
  36 at 20 weeks
  36 at 16 weeks
  36 at 12 weeks

Patients seen in July
  36 at 28 weeks
  36 at 24 weeks
  36 at 20 weeks
  36 at 16 weeks
  36 at 12 weeks

Patients seen in August
  36 at 32 weeks
  36 at 30 weeks
  36 at 28 weeks
  36 at 24 weeks
  36 at 20 weeks
  36 at 16 weeks
  36 at 12 weeks

By August, Emma will be seeing 252 patients during the month. This will take her about 63 hours. Her other hours on duty are spent according to the demands of the service. As the first deliveries are approaching, she will need to be joined by the next member of the team, Joan.

Joan, like Emma, needs to have a telephone and a car. The scheme must be explained to her very thoroughly so that she knows what she is taking on, and she and Emma need to be compatible because they will be working so closely together.

During the next couple of months, the two midwives will be seeing the following antenatal patients.

Patients seen in September
  36 at 36 weeks
  36 at 34 weeks
  36 at 32 weeks
  36 at 30 weeks

36 at 28 weeks
36 at 24 weeks
36 at 20 weeks
36 at 16 weeks
36 at 12 weeks

Patients seen in October

36 at 40 weeks
36 at 39 weeks
36 at 38 weeks
36 at 37 weeks
36 at 36 weeks
36 at 34 weeks
36 at 32 weeks
36 at 28 weeks
36 at 24 weeks
36 at 20 weeks
36 at 16 weeks
36 at 12 weeks

By October, the scheme will be fully operational and Elizabeth, the third midwife, will join the team. Like her colleagues, she needs a telephone and a car and needs to be enthusiastic about the scheme.

The three midwives are now seeing 432 antenatal patients a month. They arrange their clinics as follows:

Monday: One midwife

12 patients seen between 13.00h and 16.00h. 12 patients seen between 18.30h and 21.30h.

Wednesday: Three midwives

24 patients seen between 09.00h and 12.00h. 24 patients seen between 13.00h and 16.00h.

Friday: Two midwives

24 patients seen between 09.00h and 12.00h. 12 patients seen between 13.00h and 16.00h.

Total of 108 patients seen during the week.

Each midwife has two days off a week. The off-duty and on-call rota for October is shown in the table.

The scheme swings into action on Monday, September 30. Joan, on call since 18.00h on Sunday evening, arrives at the hospital at 06.00h - after being phoned by emergency control - because Mrs Askew has gone into labour. She will stay with Mrs Askew until she delivers (unless anything very unusual crops up).

Elizabeth comes in at 13.00h and sees 24 patients during the afternoon and evening. At 17.00h, Joan pops down to see Elizabeth on her way home from delivering Mrs Askew, and also Mrs Brown, who came in in strong labour while Joan was in the labour ward. Joan reports that Mrs Askew and Mrs Brown very much appreciated being delivered by a midwife they knew.

Elizabeth finishes her clinic at 21.30h and goes home. She is on call tonight and is called out at 03.00h to Mrs Cook, who is in false labour; Elizabeth is home again in two hours and goes back to bed. However, at 08.00h she is called again to Mrs Devi. She stays with Mrs Devi, delivers her, and leaves for home at 16.00h. Elizabeth has now worked 18.5 hours, but Emma is only now starting her week.

A chance to liaise

During Wednesday, the three midwives see 48 patients, and have a chance to liaise with each other and to visit their postnatal patients in the wards. Before the clinic finishes, Emma is called away to Mrs Farrow, who is in labour. During the evening, Mrs Cook returns to the labour ward, this time in established labour. Emma does not finish her night's work until 02.00h, and when she leaves for home she will have worked for 16 hours.

Emma and Elizabeth both spend Thursday at home because they have no one in labour, Joan is on a day off.

On Friday, Elizabeth is called out at 04.00h to Mrs Gudka, who is delivered at 10.00h. Elizabeth then goes to join Emma doing the antenatal clinic. They see 36 patients during the day and, when they leave at 16.00h, Elizabeth is going for her weekend off; having worked 37 hours, she will carry over the three hours owing into next week.

		Off-duty days	**On-call nights**
Week one	Emma Joan Elizabeth	Monday and Tuesday Thursday and Friday Saturday and Sunday	Wednesday, Friday and Sunday Tuesday and Saturday Monday and Thursday
Week two	Elizabeth Emma Joan	Monday and Tuesday Thursday and Friday Saturday and Sunday	Wednesday, Friday and Sunday Tuesday and Saturday Monday and Thursday
Week three	Joan Elizabeth Emma	Monday and Tuesday Thursday and Friday Saturday and Sunday	Wednesday, Friday and Sunday Tuesday and Saturday Monday and Thursday
Week four		the pattern continues	

Typical off duty and on call rota

Emma is not called during Friday night but on Saturday morning she arrives at the hospital at 08.00h because one of the continuity patients, Mrs Higgins, is being induced. Emma works for 10 hours and in that time delivers Mrs Isaacs, who comes in second stage, and she also takes the baby when Mrs Higgins has a Caesarean section, and hands it to Mr Higgins for a cuddle.

Joan has spent the day at home and is on call from 18.00h. At 20.00h, the phone rings; it is the beginning of a busy night for Joan. Mrs Jenkins comes in in labour; she delivers at 04.00h. Shortly afterwards, Mrs King comes into the labour ward in labour, followed by Mrs Lo in strong labour. Joan delivers Mrs Lo at 07.00h and then stays with Mrs King, who is plodding along slowly.

By 08.00h, Joan is feeling very tired; she has now worked 44 hours during the week, so she telephones Emma, who comes and takes over from her. Mrs King has a forceps delivery at 11.00h and Emma takes her to the postnatal ward at 12.30h. Having been to see all the continuity patients in the postnatal wards, Emma goes home at 14.00h to await any calls that might come in.

Between them, the continuity midwives have seen 108 antenatal patients and they have delivered 12 patients. Emma has worked 38.5 hours, Joan 44 hours and Elizabeth 37 hours. The hours they have worked over or under will be carried forward to next week and they may find it easier to arrange their timings for a fortnight or three weeks (120 hours). The three midwives will make a point of visiting their patients in the postnatal wards - this can easily be done each time they take a newly delivered mother to the ward.

Three midwives have 21 weeks of holiday between them; they may also have about one week's sick leave each. This means we have available 5,280 hours of midwife time in a year. Of those hours, 1,716 will be taken up with antenatal clinics, which leaves 3,564 hours for labours. If 36 patients are delivered a month, this leaves an average of nearly eight hours for each labour, but it must be borne in mind that some patients will be quick to deliver and sometimes two of the continuity patients will be in labour at the same time; also, of the original 36 who booked, some will miscarry and some will be transferred to total consultant care.

Satisfaction all round

I suggest that the three midwives will be able to look after at least 468 patients antenatally and during labour. The patients will be very happy with the way they are looked after and, in fact, future patients will probably be self-selected because once word gets around, many women will choose this way to have their babies.

The system is not for women having shared care with the GP, women having domino deliveries with the community midwife or for women needing specialist care -such as diabetic mothers or those who previously had Caesarean section.

It is a very economical use of midwife time, in a way which can enhance the whole experience of childbirth for the expectant mother and father - and their child. There are obviously times when it will not work smoothly: if Emma is on holiday, Joan has flu and Elizabeth has already done 42 hours work when Mrs Ransome comes into the labour ward in labour, she will have to be delivered by the labour ward staff. But she will have had continuity of care during her antenatal period and Elizabeth will pop in and visit her postnatally in the ward.

For the three midwives, it provides the satisfaction of seeing the patient all the way through; the work will be varied, with days off here and there when no one is in labour; and the midwives will have the great satisfaction of working hard whenever they are on duty - doing real midwifery at its best.

Reference

National Childbirth Trust. (1977). *Expectations of a Pregnant Woman in Relation to her Treatment.*

Reproduced with kind permission from Nursing Mirror, November 15 1979

Our Pregnant Lady

In the first of a four-part series on possible ways of improving the continuity of care for maternity patients. Caroline Flint SRN, SCM, looks at the care through the patient's eyes

Since the publication of the Short report (second report from the Social Services Committee into perinatal and neonatal mortality) many members of the medical professions have been looking into ways of implementing the recommendations of the committee concerning continuity of care for maternity patients.

Most midwives and doctors would like to provide a greater degree of continuity than is provided at present, but given the current economic situation most professionals feel bogged down providing even a basic service, and the general feeling is that continuity of care would be more expensive than the present system, both financially and in terms of midwife time. It is thought to be 'desirable, but remote'.

Over the next three weeks I will explore the possibilities of providing a scheme giving varying degrees of continuity of care for maternity patients, with the relative economics involved.

Before I start, I think it is probably unnecessary to list the benefits of continuity of care both for the practitioner and for the patient. Most general units are trying out 'patient allocation' or the 'nursing process', and are aware of the greater satisfaction that nurses reap from being directly responsible for a few patients, thus being able to really get to know intimately those patients, and that the standard of care given to those patients actually improves when a smaller number is involved in their care.

Pleas

Most of us have heard a woman complaining 'I have saw the same person twice' during an antenatal visit; or 'I had to tell my medical history each time I went, because I always saw someone different'. Many of us have listened to pleas from Community Health Councils for more continuity in the maternity department. And many midwives know the National Childbirth Trust publication, *Expectations of a Pregnant Woman in Relation to her Treatment* which says 'I would like it if were possible to have someone around during my labour who had given me some antenatal care'.

Everyone seems to be clamouring for continuity of care, but how can we provide it, and who should be providing it? If we look at who gives most overall care to a pregnant, labouring and postnatal woman we can see that 75 per cent of women in this country are delivered by midwives, usually with no doctor present, because this is the job of midwives – to be responsible for the care of the normal labouring woman, and for the normal pregnant and postnatal woman.

Constant care

If we look at maternity care through the eyes of the woman who is receiving it, we can see who provides her with the most constant care. In the antenatal clinic she is greeted by the antenatal clinic sister (midwife); she is weighed and her blood pressure is taken by a midwife; she may have a blood sample taken (probably by a midwife); her urine sample will be tested either by an auxiliary nurse or by a student midwife; she will be taken into an examination room and asked to bare her abdomen (a midwife will do this); an obstetrician (doctor) will then come in and palpate her abdomen and tell her how her baby is lying and ask her how she is – he will tell her when to attend again; during her pregnancy she may well go once or twice to the midwives' clinic where she will be seen totally by midwives.

When our pregnant lady comes to the hospital in labour she will first ring the labour ward and will speak to a midwife who will give her advice over the phone; when she and her partner come in, she will be admitted by a midwife or a student midwife who will examine her, give her suppositories or an enema and in some hospitals will shave her; she will receive comforting help and support from the midwife while she is bathing and while she is contracting.

At some time during this admission procedure she will probably also be examined by a doctor, depending on the unit and whether the midwife suspects any abnormality; during labour this lady and her partner will have a midwife or a student midwife sitting with them throughout labour, taking recordings of the fetal heart, mother's pulse, blood pressure, contractions, urinary output and generally observing and supporting the labouring woman.

At the onset of the second stage of labour the midwife will don a sterile gown and gloves and will deliver the baby into the arms of its mother. During labour the mother may, or may not, see a doctor; if she needs stitches this will probably be done by a doctor or a medical student, although in most units midwives are now learning to suture their own patients.

After the baby is born the midwife will examine it, and will only call a paediatrician (doctor) if any abnormality is suspected; the midwife will clean up the baby, give it to the mother and at this time will also try to initiate breastfeeding. After all this the mother will be blanket-bathed – probably by a midwife, but may be by an auxiliary nurse – and she will have a cup of tea and anything in the way of food that the midwife can find in the kitchen. Throughout labour the midwife is the constant supporter and helper to both the woman in labour and her partner.

After delivery the woman and her baby will be taken to the postnatal ward by a porter accompanied by the midwife who will hand over the baby and the couple to the midwife on the postnatal ward.

Run by midwives

During her postnatal stay the woman will be examined twice a day by midwives; she will be helped to breastfeed by midwives; and she will stay in a ward run by midwives. Much of the teaching of postnatal women in the care of their babies has been taken over by nursery nurses because of the shortage of midwives, but in many units it will be the midwives or student midwives who teach breastfeeding, bottle-feeding, baby bathing and changing nappies and who will look after the general care of newly delivered mothers, supervising salt baths and rest periods.

During the postnatal period, the woman will be seen several times by the obstetric houseman (doctor) and probably once during the week by a consultant obstetrician (doctor). The baby will be examined thoroughly by a paediatrician (doctor) during its stay in hospital. Once the woman is discharged home she will be seen by a community midwife and/or a health visitor several times.

Looking at this resume of an average woman's experience of maternity care, it is clear that the bulk of week-to-week and day-to-day care is given – as it always has been – by the midwife. At present the care given by midwives is shared by as many as 20 or 30 midwives, and the woman has really no chance to get to know any one midwife on an intimate level, neither has the midwife any real chance of getting to know the women in her care really well – although many midwives make a supreme effort at achieving this, even over a short period.

It seems clear that the professionals who should be trying to achieve some degree of continuity of care are the midwives. But the big problem is, how is this to be achieved?

Dream of the ideal

Let us look at the dream of the ideal – this would be when a woman is looked after throughout her pregnancy, labour and puerperium by one person, 'her midwife'. This is the way district midwives used to work and many of them remember those days with affection. But they also remember those days with not such happy memories of being forever exhausted, working for hour after hour with no real break, having no social life and feeling under enormous pressure because they were working for too long, too much and too hard.

Our professional bodies have worked hard to achieve for us a shorter working week and many of us enjoy an active social life and would hate to regress to a pattern of work where we were always 'on duty' and everything had to be subordinated to our work, however enjoyable.

Consequently, I suggest that the dream of 'one midwife' is no longer feasible. Look at your own circle of friends and you will probably be able to count on the fingers of one hand your really close friends. I would suggest that the number of midwives providing the continuity of care should never exceed five or six, and preferably fewer.

Next week I shall outline a suggested pilot scheme which contains four midwives; the following week the suggested plan will contain six midwives; and the plan on the third week will contain more midwives, but will be extremely easy to implement.

Reproduced with kind permission from Nursing Mirror, December 2, 1981.

Emma, Joan, Liz and A.N. Other

*In the second of her four articles on continuity of care
for maternity patients, Caroline Flint, SRN, SCM, outlines scheme No. 1
involving a team of four midwives looking after 200 women a year*

Continuity of care by midwives who are known to the mother would probably enhance the childbirth experience for women, possibly improve the quality of the relationship between mother and child and perhaps reduce the perinatal mortality rate.

At the same time, midwives in this scheme will experience continuity of caring, thus enriching their job satisfaction and encouraging more midwives to stay in the profession. The scheme would enable the art of midwifery to be practised to the full and would provide an efficient, humane and probably economical maternity service.

Four midwives would work together. One would be a senior sister or nursing officer who will service the team, and act as co-ordinator and administrator. But her more important function is to work as one of the team members when anyone else is on holiday or on sick leave.

I envisage the nursing officer as being able to service two teams at a time, but this may be too much. She will need to get to know all the women being looked after by the team and they will need to get to know her.

As for the other three midwives, they will have the great advantage of knowing their off-duty for at least six months in advance – it could even be worked out for a whole year – one of the greatest causes of distress among nurses and midwives would be alleviated.

The number of maternity patients who can be looked after by this team of four midwives is 200 a year.

On any one day, two of the team members will be on duty and one will have a day off; except on one day a week when all the team will work and meet together (in this scheme this is a Wednesday).

The midwives on duty work one of the two shifts. One is on the on-call day when the midwife is on call from 07.45h –19.45h; an alternative might be from midnight to midnight.

This midwife will spend the day at home with a bleep and will be called in by the hospital when a 'scheme' patient is due to come into the hospital in labour or when a scheme patient arrives at the hospital in labour; although all the scheme patients will be asked to telephone the hospital before they arrive in labour, so that the team midwife can be there ready to greet her on her arrival in the labour ward. Thus she will only be in the labour ward when there is actually someone in labour.

If no one is in labour that day – 200 patients a year means that in any one week there should be only four women in labour – the on-call midwife will come into the unit at about 18.00h and will do postnatal nursings on any patients who are part of the scheme and will generally spend the evening with them.

When she has settled them in for the night, she will either go home, where she is on call for any scheme patients who are admitted into labour, or she will sleep in an on-call room in the unit and look after any scheme patients who are admitted in labour.

The other duty is the ante- and postnatal day, which is a straight shift from 08.00 – 16.30h. This shift is divided into two, the midwife coming into the postnatal ward from 08.00h to 01.00h to do postnatal nursings on scheme patients, to bath babies, help with feeding etc.

During the afternoon she goes to the antenatal clinic where she works for two hours and sees six patients. She will undertake the total antenatal care of each patient – and it is estimated it will take 20 minutes to see each one. She will do each patient's blood pressure, weight, urinalysis, abdominal palpation and any blood taking that is needed, and will send the patient for ultrasound scanning or any other necessary tests.

The patient will not be seen by a doctor unless the midwife has any worries about her, when she will either be asked to come back to the consultant's clinic or the midwife will bleep the registrar on call and he will see her. This midwife will go off duty at 16.30h and will have the evening free.

On Wednesday no one has a day off. One of the midwives is working an antenatal and postnatal day and will, as usual, be in the antenatal clinic for the afternoon. The midwife who is on call will come into the hospital at 16.00h and will work in the antenatal clinic for two hours before going to the postnatal ward, as long as she is not with someone in labour.

The nursing officer /senior sister and the other member of the team will work from 13.00h – 21.00h and see 32 patients. They will give talks about the scheme, and hold discussions and teaching sessions with the patients and their partners about the scheme, about pregnancy and labour in general, breathing and relaxation, breastfeeding and life with a baby. They will show films and give total antenatal care as on the other days.

It will be an opportunity for the midwives to see each other and give each other support and encouragement. One of the benefits of working so closely together will be that the midwives will become friends and be able to support each other, and even swap duties if necessary.

The midwives will work a 150-hour month (37.5 hours a week) and could care for 200 patients a year. For three weeks of each month the rota will be strictly adhered to. On the fourth week, the hours done by each midwife will be totted up and the rota adjusted accordingly.

Two teams of midwives could care for 400 patients a year – that is, six midwives and one senior sister. As far as the senior sister is concerned it might be more realistic to reckon on two senior sisters for every three teams which would mean that three teams could look after 600 patients a year using 11 trained staff. At a London teaching hospital I have recently been working in, we were usually under establishment but, even so, for every 600 patients we had 12.6 trained staff (not including any grade above sister). It might be worth considering how many trained staff below the grade of nursing officer most units employ, and how many midwives are being used for each 600 patients.

The patients

Women involved in this scheme have to be ' normal', that is, no previous obstetric complications, no diabetics and no cardiac patients should be included. But late bookers or previous defaulters might find the scheme attractive.

Patients would be invited to join the scheme at their normal booking visit – when the previous obstetric history has been ascertained in the case of multips – by a handout detailing the scheme. This stresses that the patients concerned would receive the greater part of their care from midwives and, unless any complications arose, would normally only see a doctor on booking, at 32 weeks and then from 40 weeks onwards.

The patients and their partners would be invited to meet the midwives on a Wednesday evening when all the midwives would be available to discuss the scheme. Every week, four new patients would be taken into the scheme.

153

	Monday	Tuesday	Wednesday	Thursday	Friday	Saturday	Sunday	
Week one	Joan	Liz	Joan	Emma	Liz	Emma Half-day	Joan Half-day	08.00h – 16.30h Postnatal ward (5 hrs). Antenatal clinic 2hrs (6 patients).
			Liz (8hrs) Emma (2hrs)					Antenatal clinic (further 26 patients)
	Liz	Joan	Emma	Liz	Emma	Joan	Emma	On call (07.45h – 07.45h)
	Emma	Emma		Joan	Joan	Liz	Liz	Day off
Week two	Emma	Joan	Emma	Liz	Joan	Liz Half-day	Emma Half-day	08.00h – 16.30h Postnatal ward (5hrs). A/N clinic 2hrs (six patients).
			Joan (8hrs) Liz (2hrs)					Antenatal clinic (further 26 patients)
	Joan	Emma	Liz	Joan	Liz	Emma	Liz	On call (07.45h – 07.45h)
	Liz	Liz		Emma	Emma	Joan	Joan	Day off
Week three	Liz	Emma	Liz	Joan	Emma	Joan Half-day	Liz Half-day	08.00h – 16.30h Postnatal ward (5hrs). Antenatal clinic (six patients).
			Emma (8hrs) Joan (2hrs)					Antenatal clinic (further 26 patients)
	Emma	Liz	Joan	Emma	Joan	Liz	Joan	On call (07.45h – 07.45h)
	Joan	Joan		Liz	Liz	Emma	Emma	Day off

How will the scheme work? Mrs A will come to the normal booking clinic, have her history taken and undergo a thorough medical examination. She will be given a leaflet with details of the scheme, inviting her to meet the midwives on any Wednesday evening. Let us imagine she visits on week one. She is 12 weeks pregnant. She meets midwives Liz and Emma and the senior sister, who explain the scheme to her.

Mrs A is still working and would prefer to attend after work, so an appointment is made for four weeks' time on a Wednesday evening.

When she comes this time, she will see Joan and Liz; when she comes for her appointment at 20 weeks she will see Emma and Joan; and as the weeks progress, she will get to know all three midwives and the senior sister.

If her pregnancy progresses normally, she will see the midwives throughout, except at 32 weeks when she will see a consultant obstetrician or a registrar. She will be seen again by the consultant at term.

If anything untoward should occur in her pregnancy, she will be seen by the registrar on call while she is in the building or she will be asked to come back to the consultant's clinic, depending on the circumstances.

The midwives will need to be able to initiate urine tests, ultrasound scans, urinary oestriol collections, etc. Once Mrs A has left work and is attending fortnightly or weekly, she may attend during the afternoon to see a midwife who will have plenty of time to devote to her, and be able to really get to know the midwives and they her. They will note what she hopes will happen at delivery, whether she has strong feelings about drugs, enemata, shaving, etc.

Let us imagine that Mrs A, who is a primipara, goes into labour in Monday of week one. She rings the labour ward before she comes in, so that they can contact the scheme midwife. If she goes into labour on Monday morning or afternoon, Liz will be called in because she is on call. If Mrs A goes into labour on Monday evening or during the night, Liz will already be in the hospital.

Suppose she is admitted at 02.00h Tuesday morning, Liz is called from the on-call room where she is asleep, or from home.

She is with Mrs A until 08.00h, when she is due to do the postnatal nursings, and Joan is now on call. Liz will ring Joan, and between them they will decide whether Liz stays with Mrs A, and Joan will then do the postnatal nursings, or vice versa. By now Mrs A will have formed a relationship with Liz but, on the other hand, she also knows Joan well.

It is now Tuesday morning and Liz has decided to stay with Mrs A during labour. Joan, who is on call, will come into the unit and do the postnatal nursings. Mrs A is delivered at 16.00h so Joan stays on and sees the antenatal patients. As she is on call, she then does her normal on-call duties, which involves seeing the postnatal patients.

Joan retires to the on-call room at 22.30h and falls asleep, very tired. She is called at 02.00h when Mrs B arrives at the unit in labour. She may feel too tired to take on the case, so rings Emma who is not officially on call until 07. 45h, but who realizes she may be called any time after midnight. Joan arrives on the unit, and delivers Mrs B at 09.30h and is back home by 11.00h. Midwife Emma will stay at home or go out, but always with her 'bleep'.

When Liz delivers Mrs A at 16.00h on Tuesday, she is due to go off duty. Joan arrives on the labour ward, takes over from Liz, transfers Mrs A to the postnatal ward and then starts the postnatal nursings on the other scheme patients as well as Mrs A. She will be cared for during the night by the normal ward staff. Joan will be doing postnatal nursings on Wednesday morning and Emma will be there on Wednesday evening and Thursday morning – Mrs A will know them all very well.

Mrs A booked early, but what of the woman who books late, or who has been an irregular attender at the antenatal clinics? I suggest that, for this woman, the intimacy and relaxed atmosphere these midwives could provide would help her to feel happier in the hospital environment, and she would also feel she was being treated as an individual – the waiting time for antenatal visits would be reduced and her other children would be welcomed also.

On starting the scheme, only one midwives and the senior sister, would be needed for the first five months. Let us imagine Emma starts working on the scheme in March. During this month she books four

patients a week, who are all 12 weeks' pregnant. During April she books another four patients a week and also sees 16 patients who are now 20 weeks' pregnant. In May, June and July she will do the same. In August the second team midwife will need to join the scheme, because by now the original women booked are 36 weeks' pregnant, and by the end of August the third team member needs to be employed.

During these first five months, Emma will have much spare time which can be used according to the needs of the service. By September the scheme will be fully operational with the four midwives working together. The senior sister should be employed right at the beginning of the scheme; she can also be used according to the needs of the service during the early months.

This is a suggestion for a pilot study on continuity of care. I honestly do not envisage in a unit where there are 1800 deliveries annually, nine teams of three midwives plus six senior sisters because it is too complicated and because high-risk patients need more care by doctors. On the other hand, I think if one such pilot study were conducted, a great number of ideas would surface which could influence treatment of all patients in such a unit.

It has been suggested the scheme could make other hospital staff resentful of the 'exclusive ' midwives and their 'exclusive' patients. In the same way that there is sometimes resentment towards community patients and often hesitancy in treating them because of their close relationship with their 'own' midwife, this danger needs to be faced. But it is unlikely to occur if the senior sister is a good communicator and holds frequent meetings between hospital and scheme staff, and if she really listens to suggestions from her midwives.

Reproduced with kind permission from Nursing Mirror, December 9, 1981.

Crisis at Night

Caroline Flint, SRN, SCM, outlines Scheme No. 2 in this, the third of her four-part series on the continuity of care for maternity patients. This scheme involves six midwives looking after 350 antenatal women a year and at delivery, and also attempts to solve the problem of staffing a labour ward at night

Since I have been looking into the ways of implementing continuity of care, many managers have said to me, 'Caroline, our problems are with night duty, try and do something about that as well as continuity'.

Here is a plan which goes some way to help the 'crisis at night' situation with which so many hospitals are faced. It provides a midwife in the labour ward for every night of the year, primarily to look after the patients who are under a 'continuity scheme' but also to act as a pair of hands when no continuity patients are in labour. The midwives would work a 12-hour night, or an 11-hour night if preferred, with breaks in the middle. As they will only be working for two nights, and those two nights will only fall once a week at most, this should not be too tiring for them.

They would also be on call for the 12 or 13 hours that are left during the day. These on call days would also occur only twice a week. During this time on call for any continuity patients who are in labour, they will also come into hospital for eight hours during the day to work with the midwife who is seeing the continuity patients in the antenatal clinic.

This scheme is for a team of six midwives, five of whom are on the rota and one of whom is the team leader. She fills in for any midwives who are on holiday or are sick.

During any span of 24 hours from Monday to Thursday there are three midwives on duty – the midwife on the 12-hour night shift, the midwife on call and a midwife who works exclusively in the antenatal clinic for

a span of four weeks, working a nine-hour day for four days a week.

These six midwives could, between them, look after all the antenatal care and deliver 350 babies a year. The midwives would not officially be able to nurse the patients in this scheme postnatally, but they would have enough time to visit the postnatal wards daily to see the patients they knew antenatally.

The table shows how scheme works for eight weeks with six midwives whom we will call Abigail, Barbara, Colleen, Daphne, Eva and Frances.

This scheme achieves several things.
• It gets away from the present inadequate span of duties which involves two shifts of staff being on duty in the afternoon, which is the traditional time for there to be at least to do in the hospital.
• It allows members of the continuity staff to be used as pairs of hands when the service needs them.
• It gives a midwife to the service for every night of the year.
• It gives midwives an interesting and varied way of working which, combined with more patient involvement, should increase their job satisfaction.
• It gives patients more continuity if they are among the 350 per year chosen to participate. Even if they are not, they will still have a greater chance of seeing the midwife they saw in the antenatal clinic – especially if they are admitted in labour during the night.

Frances starts the scheme. She works in the antenatal clinic from Monday to Friday and tries to interest low-risk patients in the scheme. She explains that the bulk of their care will come from midwives, not doctors. Patients who specifically want doctor-orientated care can exclude themselves.

Frances will book six or seven patients weekly so that the midwives will end up with about 350 deliveries a year. Frances will utilize her spare time by being an extra pair of hands wherever the service needs her. Over the next five months she will be joined by the other five midwives, some of whom will already be working in the hospital. With this scheme one less midwife will be needed in the antenatal clinic and on night duty. One or two less midwives will be needed on day duty in the labour ward.

Frances will look after all the antenatal patients she has booked. She will test their urine, take their blood pressure, weigh them, palpate them, give them iron tablets, send them for scans, etc. In fact, she will give them full antenatal care. If a patient needs to see a doctor, Frances can easily refer her to one. The patients will be seen by a consultant obstetrician at 32 or 36 weeks and again at term.

As the scheme goes into full operation all the midwives will become involved.

Let us look at the scheme from the point of view of two patients, Mrs Jones and Mrs Brown. We shall imagine that Mrs Jones is a primigravid lady who is 36 weeks pregnant at the beginning of the rota. Mrs Jones comes to the antenatal clinic on Monday and she sees Colleen who is in the clinic this month. She also sees Daphne because Daphne is on call from 08.00 -21.00h. Daphne spends eight hours in the antenatal clinic with Colleen unless she is called to the labour ward.

Also at the clinic that day is Mrs Brown, a multigravid lady who is 37 weeks' pregnant. She, too, sees Colleen and Daphne, who, in all, see 21 patients every day (Monday – Thursday).

Mrs Jones and Mrs Brown also come to the clinic the following Monday when they are seen by Colleen and Barbara.

When the ladies come the following Monday they are seen by Colleen and Barbara again.

During Thursday night Mrs Brown goes into labour. She is looked after by Barbara and has a baby girl at 03.00h.

Mrs Jones comes to the clinic again on Monday. She is by now 39 weeks pregnant. She is seen by Colleen and Eva.

Pops in

The following week Mrs Jones is at term so she goes to see the consultant obstetrician. He is happy with her condition and tells her to come back to see him next week. While she is in the clinic she pops in to tell the midwives what the obstetrician has said. The midwives in the clinic are Colleen and Barbara again.

The following Monday Mrs Jones sees the obstetrician again. She is 41 weeks' pregnant, her blood pressure is raised, she has

	LINE	Sun	Mon	Tue	Wed	Thur	Fri	Sat	Sun	Mon	Tue	Wed	Thur	Fri	Sat	Sun	Mon	Tue	Wed	Thur	Fri	Sat	Sun	Mon	Tue	Wed	Thur	Fri	Sat
Abigail	1	×	×	×	Day	Day	×	Night	Night	×	×	×	Day	Day	×	Night	Night	×	×	×	Day	Day	×	Night	Night	×	×	×	Day
Barbara	2	Day	×	Night	Night	×	×	×	Day	Day	×	Night	Night	×	×	×	Day	Day	×	Night	Night	×	×	×	Day	Day	×	Night	Night
Colleen	3	×	A/N	A/N	A/N	A/N	×	×	×	A/N	A/N	A/N	A/N	×	×	×	A/N	A/N	A/N	A/N	×	×	×	A/N	A/N	A/N	A/N	×	×
Daphne	4	×	Day	Day	×	Night	Night	×	×	×	Day	Day	×	Night	Night	×	×	×	Day	Day	×	Night	Night	×	×	×	Day	Day	×
Eva	5	Night	Night	×	×	×	Day	Day	×	Night	Night	×	×	×	Day	Day	×	Night	Night	×	×	×	Day	Day	×	Night	Night	×	×
Frances		Senior Sister: Filling in when necessary.																											

Key
A/N: 9 hours duty in the antenatal clinic.
× : Day off
Day: On call from 08.00h – 21.00h – in antenatal clinic for 8 hours (unless with a patient in labour)
Night: On duty from 21.00h – 08.00h (in the Labour Ward)

	LINE	Sun	Mon	Tue	Wed	Thur	Fri	Sat	Sun	Mon	Tue	Wed	Thur	Fri	Sat	Sun	Mon	Tue	Wed	Thur	Fri	Sat	Sun	Mon	Tue	Wed	Thur	Fri	Sat
Eva	1	×	×	×	Day	Day	×	Night	Night	×	×	×	Day	Day	×	Night	Night	×	×	×	Day	Day	×	Night	Night	×	×	×	Day
Abigail	2	Day	×	Night	Night	×	×	×	Day	Day	×	Night	Night	×	×	×	Day	Day	×	Night	Night	×	×	×	Day	Day	×	Night	Night
Barbara	3	×	A/N	A/N	A/N	×A/N	×	×	×	A/N	A/N	A/N	A/N	×	×	×	A/N	A/N	A/N	A/N	×	×	×	A/N	A/N	A/N	A/N	×	×
Colleen	4	×	Day	Day	×	Night	Night	×	×	×	Day	Day	×	Night	Night	×	×	×	Day	Day	×	Night	Night	×	×	×	Day	Day	×
Daphne	5	Night	Night	×	×	×	Day	Day	×	Night	Night	×	×	×	Day	Day	×	Night	Night	×	×	×	Day	Day	×	Night	Night	×	×
Frances		Senior Sister: Filling in when necessary.																											

Next Rota will be Daphne –Eva – Abigail – Barbara – Colleen
then Colleen – Daphne – Eva – Abigail – Barbara
then Barbara – Colleen – Daphne – Eva – Abigail

some ankle oedema and her cervix is 'ripe'. The obstetrician suggests that her labour should be induced on Wednesday morning and Mrs Jones agrees. She tells Abigail and Barbara what is happening and they refer to the rota and tell Mrs Jones that Colleen is on call on Wednesday and will come into the unit at 08.00h to be with Mrs Jones.

In fact, Mrs Jones goes into spontaneous labour during Tuesday night. Daphne, whose first priority is any scheme patient who is in labour, is on duty in the labour ward. She looks after Mrs Jones until 08.00h when Colleen comes to the labour ward having been called there instead of the antenatal clinic. Colleen delivers Mrs Jones' baby at 11.00h.

After she has warded Mrs Jones, Colleen goes down to the clinic to join Barbara. At 16.00h another patient from the scheme is admitted to the labour ward. Colleen is still on call until 21.00h so she looks after this lady until Abigail arrives for the night shift.

Free day
Colleen has had a long day but tomorrow she has a day off and on Saturday she is free all day before going on night duty for two nights. She has practised her midwifery skills both antenatally and in the labour ward. Because of her involvement with the patients it is likely that she will go and see them while they are in the postnatal wards.

This scheme needs efficient organization as it is more complicated than last week's scheme and the bond between the five midwives will be looser. Frances needs to be very enthusiastic and sensitive to the needs of her staff.

The scheme midwives will be utilized within the hospital thus: the two midwives in the antenatal clinic (the one who is on antenatal clinic duty and the one who is on call) are only seeing 21 patients a day. They should have time to lend a hand in the clinic when the normal clinics are in operation. Over a period, the midwife on call could be utilized in the labour ward while she is not in the antenatal clinic. On Friday, Saturday and Sunday the on call midwife is free to help out anywhere in the unit unless she has a scheme patient in labour.

In some units the midwives might decide to do straight 12-hour shifts during either night or day (as it is done in the private sector). In this case, the enclosed rota would work well over a 20-week period.

Midwives work a 37 and a half hour week over 20 weeks that is 750 hours. If the midwives work 12-hour shifts with an hour for meal breaks except for the four weeks when they are in the antenatal clinic, they will work 744 hours over a 20-week period. This takes into account the shortened meal breaks they will take if they are pushed for time, or the slight overlap they will sometimes have at the end of the shift.

This scheme could be adapted to many situations. As far as the patients are concerned I do not think it would be as enjoyable for them as last week's scheme. However, in many units this scheme might be easier to implement.

Next week's scheme is very easy to implement – it uses more staff, but nearly all patients would be included.

Reproduced with kind permission from the Nursing Mirror, December 16 1981.

Small is Intimate

In the last of her four-part series on continuity of care for maternity patients, Caroline Flint, SRN, SCM. explains Scheme No. 3, which involves dividing a large maternity unit into smaller and more intimate sections

This scheme was suggested to me by Vera Mitchell, a community midwife on the south coast. Her idea is to divide the care in a big consultant unit into manageable numbers so that patients get to know the midwives who are looking after them throughout their care. This is achieved by attaching midwives to each consultant.

For this scheme we must imagine a large obstetric unit delivering 3,000 babies a year. In the unit there are four obstetric teams under the overall supervision of four obstetricians.

When we are dealing with 3.000 women a year, probably about 500 will be in need of total obstetric care - i.e., the women with poor obstetric histories, diabetic women, women with infertility problems and other problems. These women will need to see the consultant or registrar at every visit antenatally, will need to have their intrapartum care supervised by them.

For these women there will need to be a skeleton staff of midwives in the antenatal clinic and in the labour ward, probably in the region of only one midwifery sister and one staff midwife at any one time, probably with a nursing auxiliary on hand in the labour ward. Probably a further 100 women would be looked after by the community midwives either as 'domino' cases or home confinements. Thus we are left with 2,400 potentially 'normal' pregnant women a year.

Apart from the skeleton staff on the labour ward and in the antenatal clinic, all the other midwives work in the wards. There are four antenatal/postnatal wards - one for each consultant - or there are two antenatal/postnatal wards divided in half.

The midwives are attached to a consultant obstetrician, who look after his patients almost exclusively - I say almost because there are always times when the best schemes fall down and a situation may arise when all Mr A's midwives are down with flu - but to all intents and purposes each midwife would work with one obstetric team. She would stay on the ward for a long period - at least a year - and she would rotate as far as night duty was concerned. All antenatal care would be carried out on the ward and would be done by midwives except, probably, for two visits to the antenatal clinic to see the obstetrician.

The midwives would work normal hours: 07.45-16.30h; 12.30h-21.30h; or 21.00h-08.00h. The antenatal patients could be seen during the overlap period in the afternoon. With 2,400 deliveries a year, each team would look after 600 women a year and would need to see 25 or 26 women daily, antenatally - this does not include Saturday or Sunday, but it could.

Two midwives could examine patients between 13.00h and 16.00h. If each patient was given 15 minutes, they would see 24 patients during that time. The advantage to women being seen in this way is that they would get to know the midwives, the postnatal ward and other women who are in-patients; they could discuss with women who had been delivered what labour was like, and they could get the 'feel' of hospital.

When a woman comes into the hospital in labour, a midwife off her ward is called to look after her. By the time she has been coming to the ward for 11 visits the labouring woman should know most of the midwives, would be looked after in labour by one of the ward midwives and then postnatally by the same midwives.

Ideally, each ward would have 15 to 16 midwives rotating to provide three on early shift; two on evening shift; and three during the night. The labour ward would need seven midwives to provide two on early shift; one on late shift and two at night. The antenatal clinic would need three midwives to provide a skeleton service of two midwives at any one time.

The 16 midwives on each ward would work the same shifts they are working at the moment - the only difference being that they would always work on that ward and they would not rotate to any other part of the hospital.

For patients, the difference would be that their antenatal care is carried out in the ward where they spend their postnatal period - except for their visits to see their consultant obstetrician.

When patients are in labour, one of their consultant's midwives will be called from the ward to look after them - midwives will be undertaking all aspects of maternity care, they will be more satisfied with their jobs and they will have the satisfaction of getting to know their patients well.

From the patients' point of view, it is much less satisfactory to try to get to know 16 midwives than a smaller number, but this scheme would be so easy to implement that it might be the scheme of choice for many units.

Having now documented three different - but all entirely feasible - methods of achieving some continuity of care in a maternity unit, I hope I have been able to show that, contrary to most opinion, continuity does not require more staff then our present system - in fact, in some instances it utilizes staff more efficiently.

Reproduced with kind permission from Nursing Mirror, December 23/30 1981

Where Have We Gone Wrong?

Health care for pregnant women has been much criticized recently, although midwives have been doing their best to provide a satisfactory service. Caroline Flint begins a nine-part series on antenatal clinics with an investigation into why this situation has arisen

For the past two years antenatal clinics have been under attack. The Spastics Society started with their film *Feeling Special* and they were followed by the Short report, Esther Rantzen in *That's Life*, the National Childbirth Trust in *Change in Antenatal Care*, the Spastics Society in *Who's Holding the Baby Now?* and countless local newspapers and consumers.

Many of those working in antenatal clinics are doing their best to provide an adequate service for too many women in overcrowded buildings with two few staff. Many of us are aware of the criticisms and indeed often feel that they are justified - but what can we do to improve our service given the present cuts in NHS spending?

This series is for you and your ideas - suggestions from those working in the field with ideas that have worked for them - ideas to be floated that have never yet been tried, ideas from women going through the system and women who have already been through it. So whoever you are, student nurse to district nursing officer, please get your pad and pen and start sending your ideas to Caroline Flint c/o *Nursing Mirror*.

The aim of this series is to improve delivery of antenatal care by looking at ideas and practices, thinking through new ideas and suggestions, thinking about the care we are giving a 'shake up'. We may decide afterwards that what we are doing is best in the circumstances or we may decide to try something different. Let us try to define the most common problems.

The impersonality of the experience at a time when women are feeling especially emotionally vulnerable. The Short report talks about the 'cattle truck atmosphere of antenatal clinics where there is little privacy, little dignity'. A woman in *The British Way of Birth* says: 'I felt I was wasting everyone's time...theirs and mine. I was kept waiting for up to two and a half hours to have less than two minutes with a doctor who talked to me with his back to me'.

Change in Antenatal Care says: 'The expectant mother is treated as the passive object of management, who is fed into the system and whose progress through it from point to point is controlled as if she had no wishes or preferences of her own.'

Long waiting times

Change in Antenatal Care says: 'Waiting times are long, often two hours or more, and sometimes exceed three hours, in surroundings which are often extremely uncomfortable and frequently depressing. Few hospitals provide anything for women to do except wait.'

A woman in *The British Way of Birth* says: 'I never waited less than one and a half hours and on two occasions I left after two hours without being examined, to catch transport.'

Short consultation times with obstetricians

Change in Antenatal Care says: 'Contact with an obstetrician is restricted to one or two minutes. To many women this seems the whole point of the visit, and all the planning and waiting are directed towards this moment. But for the most the visit culminates in only a brief laying on of hands by a member of the obstetric team who may have no more idea of who the person is he is examining than she does of him. It is not surprising that women feel disappointed when they are in and out of the examination room in a matter in minutes and have no opportunity for discussion or voicing anxieties.'

A woman in *The British Way of Birth* says: 'The clinic is very overcrowded, you can be waiting for up to two and a half hours just to see the doctor for two minutes.'

Lack of continuity of care

Evidence from the Spastics Society quoted in the Short report says: 'I think this is what women complain about most: they do not have continuity of care, which they want very much during their antenatal visits but certainty during labour and delivery.'

This leads on to a recommendation in the Short report: 'We recognize the difficulties of providing continuity of care throughout pregnancy and labour but consider that a measure of it can be obtained by better organization.'

A woman in *The British Way of Birth* says: 'I never saw the same doctor twice, they were examining you as if you were part of a car.'

Change in Antenatal Care says: 'There is almost a complete absence of continuity of care and each time she attends a woman may see different, anonymous faces and also be given conflicting information and advice which leads to anxiety and confusion.'

If these are the problems, we could define our aims as:
• to help women to feel special when they come to the clinic, so that they feel that they are valued personally and that the staff are interested in them as individuals, and for the woman to feel that she has some control over the situation.
• to cut down the waiting time in clinics and to make any waiting that cannot be avoided into a positive experience;
• to enable the actual consultation to be longer, more meaningful for the woman, and for her to feel that she is being seen as a person not as a 'pregnant-shaped container'
• to attempt to provide the same staff each time the woman visits the clinic.

First let us look at the antenatal clinics in most hospitals and see the great variety of antenatal care that exists, even in the same town.

The first antenatal visit a woman makes to the hospital varies enormously from clinic to clinic. Some women 'book' their bed over the phone, some send their doctors letter to the hospital, some women have to appear in person and some hospitals 'book' beds according to a co-operation card sent in by the woman's GP, some hospitals have a 'documentation clinic' when women can arrive any time between 13.00 and 15.00h on Tuesday and Thursday afternoon

Different regimes

Some antenatal clinics hold a booking clinic at a different time from the ordinary 'follow-on' clinic sessions. Other clinics incorporate new patients in with the ordinary follow-on patients. Some booking clinics consist of midwives taking medical and obstetric histories from the women and then the women return a week or fortnight later to see one of the doctors.

In some clinics the midwives also weigh the women at this first visit, take their blood pressure, test their urine, take their blood and palpate them – even though nothing is palpable before 12 weeks, this gets the woman used to having her abdomen felt. In this way the woman is introduced to the midwife's role and it gives the midwife the opportunity to pick up anyone who is booking late or is very large for dates. Some booking clinics consist of a three-and-half hour marathon where the patient has a medical and obstetric history taken by a midwife. Then the prospective mother is weighed, measured, produces a midstream specimen of urine, sees a dietician, physiotherapist, social worker and health visitor. She has a blood sample taken, has a full medical examination (including vaginal examination and cervical smear) from a doctor and then goes on tour of the obstetric unit.

Some antenatal clinics expect all the women to undress and sit in rows in identical hospital dressing gowns.

Some antenatal clinics do not ask the women to undress. Others ensure that the woman has talked to the doctor who is going to examine her, with her clothes on and sitting up in a chair, before she is asked to undress for her physical examination.

At some clinics vaginal examinations are performed at booking (to detect pelvic abnormalities or growths, to determine the size of the pregnancy and to perform a cervical smear). Sometimes clinics do not perform a vaginal examination because the policy is that the fetal head is the best indicator of pelvic adequacy. Other clinics do the examination at 36 weeks when the action of circulating progesterone makes it a far more comfortable procedure for the pregnant woman.

The fascinating aspect of this huge variety is that each clinic considers its procedures to be the 'right way', even though a sister hospital in the next street carries out a completely different regime with apparently similar obstetric outcomes in an apparently similar population.

Sheila Kitzinger in her *Women as Mothers* suggests that these are rituals that we subject the woman to: 'The organization of many antenatal clinics incorporates procedures which many patients find humiliating . . . Patients wait, with their specimens, in rows and dressed in white hospital smocks, as they are slowly processed through the clinic system. . . Naked from the waist down,

she lies flat while a group of men form round her lower end and her abdomen and her vagina is uncomfortably and sometimes painfully prodded and explored . . . her private parts are referred to as 'the vulva', 'the bladder', 'the perineum', 'the uterus', thus depersonalizing them . . . In the modern hospital this is our own ceremonial *rite de passage* into motherhood. It involves separation from 'normal' people going about their everyday lives; taking over by agencies outside the woman's control; investigation and assessment involving exposure of the most intimate parts of the body to men and strangers; and subjection to alarming and sometimes painful procedures at which she must not flinch because 'it is for the sake of the baby'. Only after these rites of separation and humiliation does society remake her as a mother.

Kitzinger is not the only person to question what antenatal care is really about. In a paper questioning the efficacy of conventional antenatal care given by Sally MacIntyre at the 1980 research and the midwife conference in Glasgow entitled 'Interaction in antenatal clinics' , MacIntyre quoted from her questioning of pregnant and postnatal women and found that 50 per cent of women were neutral about the supposed benefits of antenatal care and a further 25 per cent thought that their antenatal care had been useless – leaving only 25 per cent who had ben able to detect any positive benefits from their antenatal clinic visits. Her study also showed that more than half the patients seeing their consultant obstetrician had consultations of 2.9 minutes only.

In *The British Way of Birth* a woman says: 'Hospital examinations were sometimes so basic that they could have been done at the GPs with less all round expense, time and bother to all parties'.

In the *Journal of the Royal Society of Medicine*, Chamberlain says: 'It is still worth trying to re-examine current ideas and not to accept blindly that every procedure is bound to be helpful. Everything should be assessed periodically to see if it is effective and being used efficiently. Such scrutiny may improve both care of the individual patient and the more general use of facilities. In many ways antenatal care is a good subject for such an assessment'.

In *The Lancet*, Marion Hall questioned the productivity of routine antenatal care in a paper entitled '*Is routine antenatal care worthwhile?*' and outlined a scheme in which women without special problems are seen in the antenatal clinic only five times, at 12 weeks for booking, at 22 weeks to detect multiple pregnancy, at 30 weeks, 36 weeks and again at term.

Whether antenatal clinic visits are sometimes beneficial, always beneficial, or rarely beneficial is a different debate but those of us who work in antenatal clinics need to make clinic visits something that women enjoy and look forward to, so that if in the future the clinic visit is shown not to be as beneficial as we have always accepted, at least the women will feel that they have spent happy times with us.

References

Boddy, K., Parboosingh, J., Shepard, C. *A Schematic Approach to Prenatal Care*. Department of Obstetrics and Gynaecology, Edinburgh University.

Boyd, C., Sellers, L. (1982). *The British Way of Birth*. Pan Books.

Chamberlain, G. (1978). 'A re-examination of antenatal care'. *Journal of the Royal Society of Medicine*, 71, September.

Chng, P., MacGillivray, I. (1980). 'An audit of antenatal care: The value of the first antenatal visit.' *British Medical Journal*, 281, November 1.

DHSS (1980). *Perinatal and Neonatal Mortality*. Second report from the Social Services Committee: HMSO.

Hall, M., Chng,P., MacGillivray, I. (1980). 'Is routine antenatal care worthwhile?'. *The Lancet*, July 12.

Kitzinger, S. (1978). *Women as Mothers*. Fontana Books.

MacIntyre, S. (1980). 'Interaction in antenatal clinics.' Paper given at Research and the Midwife Conference, Glasgow.

National Childbirth Trust (1981). 'Change in antenatal care'. Report from working party set up for the NCT by Sheila Kitzinger.

Oakley, A. (1981). *From here to Maternity. Becoming a Mother*. Pelican Books.

Spastics Society (1981). *Who's Holding the Baby now?* July.

Spastics Society. *Feeling special*. A film about care before birth, produced by Randel Evans Productions Ltd. directed by Nigel Evans.

Reproduced with kind permission from Nursing Mirror, November 24 1982.

Get Off the Conveyor Belt

Many pregnant women are treated as medical cases when they attend their antenatal clinic. They feel like 'objects of passive management' at a time when it is important for them to feel special. In the second of her series, Caroline Flint describes how they tackle this problem at her clinic

How can we help a woman feel special when she comes to the antenatal clinic, how can we help her feel valued personally and how can we help the woman to feel that she has some control over her pregnancy, her labour and her baby?

How do women feel when they come to our clinic? How can we find out how they feel? Do the women feel like 'passive objects of management', like the women reported in the National Childbirth Trust's *Change in Antenatal Care*, or do they enjoy coming?

One of the best ways to find out how the clinic appears to the women using it, is to have a friend who is going through the system. But try to resist the temptation of making it extra nice for her. Then quiz her on impressions afterwards. One successful way we found was to get a staff midwife to come in her ordinary clothes and to join the women in the clinic. Afterwards she jotted down her impressions and we gained a revealing insight into the running of the clinic. And the staff midwife also benefited from the experience and it helped her to view her clients with new eyes.

But the most obvious way of finding out what women think of our service is to ask them. Asking directly may not elicit a full answer because if you are obviously making an effort to improve the antenatal clinic the women will be reluctant to hurt your feelings by telling you how it really appears to them.

If you are making a tremendous effort to improve your antenatal clinic it will also be hard for you to listen to what the women are really saying because you have so much emotional energy invested in the clinic and how it runs.

Perhaps the easiest way of finding out how women view the clinic is through a questionnaire. This must be anonymous - no names and no hospital numbers on it - and the questions must be carefully worded.

For example, it is difficult to answer the following question in anything but a positive way: 'We have recently tried to improve our antenatal clinic, are you finding the waiting time is shorter than it was?'

Much more information will be gathered by open questions, such as;

• Please list what you enjoy about your visits to the antenatal clinic;

• Please list what you dislike about the antenatal clinic;

• Please write down any suggestions you have to help us make the clinic better for you.

• To find out how long women are usually waiting ask;

• What time was your appointment?

• What time did you arrive?

• What time were you seen by the doctor or midwife?

The other easy trap to fall into is the 'it's better than it was' syndrome. The clinic will probably be improving all the time. You have reduced the waiting time from three hours to one hour; you have made the clinic an interesting place to visit. It is definitely a better service than it was, but this is irrelevant to the woman who comes to the clinic for the first time. This is how an antenatal clinic is to her and she does not know that it can be any different. She sees the clinic as 'here and now'.

Because of this, 'old customers' can be unhelpful because they will say 'Oh sister, it's so much better than it was last year/when I had my Danny/when my sister came'. Although this is music to your ears it can blind you to the here and now that new clients see.

Other people who can help clinic staff gain insight into the actual service are members of the local community health council. The CHC may be willing to conduct a survey in the clinic or place an observer there to see what is actually happening. Organizations, such as the National Childbirth Trust or the Association for Improvements in the Maternity Services, can often help in this way too.

A questionnaire does not pick up the feelings of less literate women, but often the more articulate woman will voice common feelings.

Ann Oakley, in her two books *From Here to Maternity* and *Women Confined*, outlines very clearly what women think about their antenatal care. One woman says 'It's your first experience, and you feel as though you're the only one in the world having a baby. I think they should make you feel as though you're a little bit important.'

How can we do this? How can we help women to feel special?

Helping a woman to feel special starts before she visits the clinic. At St George's we send every woman a welcoming letter before she comes to the booking clinic. In this letter we welcome her to the hospital, detail all that will happen in the booking clinic and ask her to give us any suggestions and comments to improve our service.

We do this so that each woman can visualize what will happen at the booking clinic. She can discuss it with her partner and if she decides that she does not want to participate in something that we have on offer, she can decide about it and prepare herself mentally for her visit.

Many women attending an antenatal clinic will never have been inside a hospital before. A first-time attender is probably apprehensive, nervous and feels very unsure of herself. She also may be embarrassed - it might be the first time she has acknowledged her pregnancy.

Generally people can only listen to someone talking for 20 minutes and they take in perhaps 50 per cent of what has been said. Because of this we also need to realise that pregnant women, who are particularly self-absorbed, sometimes seem to take in less and even less when they are frightened and nervous?

So at her first visit, we have a woman who is frightened and who will not take in a great deal of what we are saying to her. I would be grateful for your suggestions about how you deal with this problem.

At our clinic we sit down with the women when they arrive and welcome them collectively. Then we go through what happens at the booking clinic again. We also tell them that we are trying to improve our clinics and that we need their comments and suggestions in order to do that. Then we indicate who is here for the first time and welcome back women who have been before. The 'old-timers' are invited to tell the first-timers what it is like having a baby in our hospital. During this time we aim to get the women talking to each other and so set up a peer group who will recognize each other every time they come to the clinic. If a woman can make a friend at her antenatal clinic we will have given her a great gift. The friends women make in their first pregnancy often remain close friends for much of their adult life.

The way that we usually feel special is when other people know us as an individual and when they are interested in us as an individual. We incorporate this principle into our booking clinic by trying to get to know each women as she comes to us. When the midwife takes a booking history we ask each women several questions about how she feels about her pregnancy, childbirth in general and what specific anxieties or hopes she has for this pregnancy.

In this way each woman has an opportunity to have a longish talk with the midwife. Ideally, of course, one midwife would follow one particular woman all the way through her pregnancy - but we are still working towards this.

Another way we try to show that we recognize each woman's individuality is by having a 'hostess' at the entrance of the follow-on clinics. The hostess is usually the sister, who greets each woman as she enters and in our clinic we go through the woman's notes with her and decide who she would like to see this visit.

Many woman become very attached to one midwife or one doctor and request to see that person at each visit. Sometimes women take a dislike to one midwife or one doctor and specifically request not to see that person. By having a discussion with the sister, each woman feels that she has some control over what happens to her at each clinic visit. *Change in Antenatal Care* says 'Women feel they are on a conveyor belt which must be kept moving at all costs.' Not only do women hate the conveyor belt type of clinic management but so do midwives. When you have taken 45 women's blood pressures you begin to have ringing in the ears. However well-intentioned the midwife or nurse is by the time she gets to woman number 45, her smile has begun to waver and all she is longing for is her lunch break. This applies to the nurse who tests the urine samples or the one who weighs a long queue of patients. How horrendous for any woman to be one of a long line of women being weighed - a touchy measurement at the best of times - but to be weighed in public is very embarrassing.

To overcome this we have copied the GP's surgery where everything is done in the one room. Each woman is weighed, has her blood pressure taken, has her abdomen palpated in the same room. When the system works at its best, the same person does all these procedures to the woman. This also lengthens the time she has to talk to her attendant, because she will be chatting to her while she is being weighed or having her blood pressure taken. This system also means the medical attendant whether doctor or midwife will be able to get to know each woman a little better.

This week I have explored a few ways that we could perhaps try to make the antenatal clinic a nicer place for women. Now I am waiting for your comments and suggestions. The last article in this series will be devoted to your ideas.

References

Boddy, K., Parboosingh, J., Shepard, C. *A Schematic Approach to Prenatal Care.* Department of Obstetrics and Gynaecology, Edinburgh University.

Boyd, C., Sellers, L. (1982). *The British Way of Birth.* Pan books.

Chamberlain, G. (1978). 'A re-examination of antenatal care'. *Journal of the Royal Society of Medicine*, 71, September.

Chng, P., MacGillivray, I. (1980). 'An audit of antenatal care: The value of the first antenatal visit'. *British Medical Journal*, 281, November .

DHSS (1980). *Perinatal and Neonatal Mortality.* Second report from the Social services Committee: HMSO.

Hall, M., Chng, P., MacGillivray, I. (1980). 'Is routine antenatal care worthwhile?'. *The Lancet*, July 12.

Kitzinger, S. (1978). *Women as Mothers.* Fontana Books.

MacIntyre, S. (1980). 'Interaction in antenatal clinics'. Paper given at Research and the Midwife conference, Glasgow.

National Childbirth Trust (1981). 'Change in antenatal care'. Report from working party set up for the NCT by Sheila Kitzinger.

Oakley, A. (1980). *Women Confined Towards a Sociology of Childbirth.* Martin Robertson and Co. LTD.

Oakley, A. (1981). *From here to Maternity. Becoming a Mother.* Penguin Books.

Spastics Society (1981). *Who's Holding the Baby now?*

Reproduced with kind permission from Nursing Mirror, December 1 1982.

Make it Worth the Wait

Mothers-to-be often feel exasperated at the amount of time they spend waiting to be seen at antenatal clinics. Caroline Flint discusses how waiting times can be reduced by a sensible appointment system and how any time spent waiting can be filled constructively

Waiting times in hospital antenatal clinics have always been notoriously long, but is there any way to improve them? All the reports I have referred to previously have highlighted the horrors of the waiting times that women are subjected to. In *The British Way of Birth*, 1,880 women (37 per cent) said that they had to wait between one and two hours to be seen in their antenatal clinics. One woman said 'An absolutely appalling, unreasonable waiting time.'

Change in Antenatal Care, from the National Childbirth Trust working party, says 'Waiting times are long, often two hours or more, and sometimes exceed three hours in surroundings which are often extremely uncomfortable and frequently depressing.'

Have you found any good ways to shorten your waiting times?

Last week I described a questionnaire that women coming to the clinic can be asked to fill in. This asks what time their appointment is, what time they actually arrived and what time they were actually seen. Of course the information obtained is valuable, but perhaps it is even more helpful to have a volunteer in the clinic for about three or four weeks whose sole function is to jot down the times when women are seen by a doctor or midwife and to tally the appointment times to those realistic times rather than to an imagined number of 'how many we should be able to see in such and such a time'. This means that the appointment book will not look so neat.

A realistic system means that women coming to the clinic will not have to wait around until the doctors arrive. And women will not be arriving in droves while the clinic stops for a coffee break.

Having achieved a realistic appointment system, you must anticipate that it will not last for ever. The system should be reviewed at least every six months and maybe more often. Every time a doctor changes it means a slight adjustment in the way the clinic works.

Intention	Reality
08.30h 10 patients	08.30h 0 patients
08.45h 10 patients	08.50h 2 patients
09.00h 10 patients	09.05h 8 patients
09.15h 10 patients	09.25h 10 patients

Last week I was shocked that the clinic which we had designated as 'most impressive' in our minds as far as waiting times were concerned six months ago, has once again degenerated into an upturned anthill - so constant vigilance is needed!

Once midwives are used for seeing pregnant women the waiting time in a clinic is immediately reduced because of the full utilization of staff.

The Short report says 'We have also recommended that more use should be made of experienced midwives who could relieve much of the load on obstetricians by providing part of the antenatal care for the "low risk" mother.'

It continues 'Steps should be taken to make better use of the skills of the midwife in maternity care - particularly in the antenatal clinic and labour ward, where they should be given greater responsibility for antenatal care of women with uncomplicated pregnancies.'

In most antenatal clinics the midwives are *there*, and their great advantage is that no one has to wait for them to arrive. When women are waiting to be seen, the midwives can see them immediately and usually in a very satisfactory manner. In the NCT report *Change in Antenatal Care* the working party recommends 'We call for a new recognition of midwifery. A midwife is *fully qualified to give total antenatal care*. In the long-term we should like to see midwifery extended to concern with women's health generally, as in some women's clinics in the USA, so that there is a continuing relationship before, during and after pregnancy.'

In many clinics, midwives weigh women, take their blood pressures, give them certificates of expected confinement, test urine, act as chaperones or as the Royal College of Midwives said in their evidence to the Short committee 'the midwife is there as his (the doctor's) handmaiden to support him'.

It is time the midwives did a full consultation with women in their clinics. Expertise is being lost and confidence in the midwifery profession is fairly low, but experience is only gained with practice. The way we have gained confidence in our midwifery skills is by the way we run our 'midwives clinic' - but more about that next week.

As well as a 'midwives clinic' we also have midwives seeing women in all our consultant's clinics. This gives the midwives confidence that the doctors are at hand if they have any worries. It also gives the consultants confidence because they feel that their patients are not disappearing from their care and that if the midwives detect anything worrying they will immediately call for help.

One of the first things we did at St George's was to look at how we were utilizing the available space. We listed the number of consultation rooms and the number of people using them. It might be worth taking a fresh look at how you are using the space in your own clinic. If you have eight consultation rooms, eight doctors or midwives are using them and seeing eight women at one time then you are utilizing them to the full. But if you have eight consultation rooms, only four medical attendants who skip between two rooms each, then you are using four of your rooms as waiting rooms. Next week I will show how the potential for a much poorer consultation is increased because of this.

Having looked at reducing the overall waiting time in the antenatal clinic, it is still obvious that some women will have to wait sometimes. As the NCT's *Change in Antenatal Care* states 'Few hospitals provide anything for women to do *except* wait'. What facilities can we provide with limited budgets and limited staff?

We have noticed a significant difference in the level of conversation in our clinic when we have the chairs arranged in rows (very little conversation) and when we arranged the chairs in small circles (much more conversation).

Sometimes we label each circle of chairs with the names of surrounding districts - Tooting, Streatham or Wimbledon, and we suggest that women sit in their own district in the hope that they will strike up a conversation with someone who lives near them.

Of course, this is much easier if a volunteer or staff member goes round to each circle in turn and attempts to introduce the women to each other. If a pregnant mother can leave her antenatal clinic having made a friend by the end of her pregnancy, the clinic will have given her something of enormous value - even if later research shows that her actual antenatal care is of limited value.

Refreshments while waiting, make a clinic feel much more homely and are needed by women who have travelled a long way to attend the clinic. Most hospitals have volunteers who give sterling service in the assorted clinics. At booking clinics it is very friendly if the midwife who takes the woman's history can sit down with her and have a cup of tea with her.

Any clinic can find a small space for children to play in, if ex-patients can be persuaded to come back and look after the children and donate toys, paints and so on the atmosphere in the clinic is immediately improved. The children's play area has more value than is immediately apparent.

Its primary function is, of course, to entertain the children while their mothers receive their antenatal care. This lowers the noise level in the clinic and makes the noises happy noises rather than bored noises. The presence of children being played with, is educational for 'primips' who can learn much by seeing how the children are handled. At St George's we are blessed because we have someone who runs a nursery school to run our playroom.

With her expertise she is able to show how to stimulate and educate children - this is helpful to both the women waiting in the clinic and the volunteer helpers. The other benefit of the playroom is that it acts as a meeting place for the helpers who often have new babies and can be feeling quite lonely and isolated.

In hospitals, we often do not appreciate the importance of notices. In any hospital one can also see old signs that the staff no longer notice because they have been there so long. It is worth going round and checking that the lavatories are clearly labelled, that the public phone is indicated and that all the rooms with doctors and midwives in, are clearly labelled with their names.

This prevents women feeling that they are sitting in the wrong place and that they have been forgotten (a horrible and common feeling in out-patients clinics). If a woman has discussed with the sister/hostess, that she is going to see Dr Jones or Midwife Cooper she feels much more secure if she is waiting outside a room that is labelled Dr Jones or Midwife Cooper. This need not cost anything, we use yellow card - left over from X-rays which the X-ray department keep for us - written on with big letters in thick felt tip pen.

Many people are used to a television being on in a corner of their room. There are many excellent films and videos available for screening in a corner of the antenatal clinic. For no cost they can give women an enormous amount of pleasure and they can have great educational value as well. Usually a projector can be borrowed from the local health education department. We now have the luxury of a daylight screen, but originally we used to project our films inside a cupboard with women sitting outside it.

The antenatal clinic is the ideal place to do antenatal teaching Often subjects crop up with a question asked by one of the women waiting and this can lead to a discussion. If a midwife (with a fairly loud voice) can be spared to do antenatal teaching in the clinic this can transform the waiting time into a period of interest and usefulness.

Other departments also can be a source of teaching: dieticians may put on a display of iron rich foods, or fibre in food; physiotherapists can be encouraged to talk about and demonstrate posture during the clinic and the local library service can be asked to bring selections of books on pregnancy, childbirth, sex education for siblings, or on useful books for toddlers.

Reproduced with kind permission from Nursing Mirror, December 8 1982

More Than a Laying on of Hands

Consultations with doctors in antenatal clinics are often rushed, leaving the women feeling disappointed that they have not had the opportunity to ask questions about their pregnancies. Caroline Flint describes how the system was changed at her clinic to allow more meaningful and better consultations for both the women and the doctors

Women often complain bitterly about the shortness of their consultations with the doctors at the antenatal clinics. In *The British Way of Birth* one woman says 'It feels like a factory in the hospital. You actually spend a total of two minutes with the doctor so it all seems a waste of time.'

The National Childbirth Trust's working party report *Change in Antenatal Care* states: 'For most the visit culminates with a brief laying on of hands by a member of the obstetric team who may have no more idea of whom the person is he is examining than she does of him. It is not surprising that women feel disappointed when they are in and out of the examination room in a matter of minutes and have no opportunity for discussion or for voicing anxieties'.

We have already looked at ways of utilizing midwifery skills so that more women see midwives, thus freeing the doctors for a longer and more meaningful consultation with fewer women. But let us look at how the clinic is arranged so that the woman can spend the maximum amount of time with her medical attendant.

One of the most dehumanizing of experiences is waiting in a queue to be weighed publicly or queuing to have one's blood pressure taken. Even though these procedures may appear to streamline the clinic I suggest that it actually hampers the consultation with the doctor.

Women attending clinics have many questions to ask and many comments to make.

If the women queue have measurements of weight, blood pressure and urine the questions that crop up at that time remain unanswered because it seems useless to ask someone who is weighing 120 women. Women usually wait to ask the person who palpates them. If the person who usually weighs them is a midwife, perhaps her skills could be better used seeing women for a complete antenatal consultation.

Quality

At St George's Hospital; we made a radical difference to the quality of consultations when we bought scales for each consulting room so that women are always weighed in a room with a doctor present. This initiates conversation about how the woman is eating, she also has her blood pressure taken at the doctor's desk so that she is sitting down at the same level as the doctor which encourages her to talk to him or her. Only after she has had the opportunity to chat to the medical attendant does she lie down on the couch to be palpated. We are trying to imitate the GP's surgery where everything is done in one room and women have the opportunity to talk all the way through the consultation.

When the doctor sees the woman walk into the room he or she can ascertain many points that would not be picked up with the woman lying down throughout the consultation. The way a woman walks, holds herself, looks, shows if she has any skeletal abnormalities, if she is depressed, if she is feeling beaten, if she is poor, undernourished or if she feels happy and well.

This description explains why I suggested, last week, that the quality of the consultation is decreased when a doctor uses two rooms because he or she misses so much when a patient is only seen while she is lying down.

Disadvantaged

Horizontal women find it more difficult to talk, to negotiate, to remember what questions they wanted to ask. Women lying down are very disadvantaged if they only see their medical attendants in this position. I believe that we shall never achieve excellent and satisfactory antenatal care as far as our patients are concerned until we start by seeing all women sitting up, in their normal clothes and at the same physical level as the doctor.

Midwives seem to do this quite automatically, and it is interesting to see that when women are used to having a choice between a consultation with a midwife or with a doctor they often opt for the midwife because they know there will be more opportunity to talk and ask questions.

The quality of the consultation is improved when it is accepted by all medical attendants that an integral part of obstetric care is how a woman feels about what is happening to her. This is most easily introduced by use of the nursing process in midwifery, when women are given an opportunity to discuss how they feel about their pregnancy and labour and their forthcoming role as a mother.

When a woman knows her medical attendant the quality of the consultation is much better. And the medical attendant also finds enormous pleasure seeing women and already knowing their names. Continuity of care is difficult to achieve in most antenatal clinics in the way that we run them at the moment. But we achieve a quite a high level of continuity in our midwives' clinic by allocating women to the same midwife each time they come. Midwife Omari has red stickers on her patients' notes, Midwife Thomas has green. Each midwife has 15 minute appointments and so each women is given a realistic appointment always with the same midwife.

This seems to be more difficult to achieve at the consultants' clinics when we are dealing with far more women. But we achieve some degree of continuity by the sister/hostess greeting each woman as she arrives - going through her notes with her, and asking her whom she would like to see this week. Women then have the opportunity to say 'Can I see Doctor X, I always see him' or 'Can I see Midwife Y, she wanted to know about my daughter's rash'.

Some clinics must have conquered this problem by now, have you? Please write and let us know - all ideas gratefully received.

Reproduced with kind permission from Nursing Mirror, December 15 1982

Continuity of Care

Caroline Flint explains why mothers-to-be need to see the same midwives and consultants throughout their antenatal care. She describes how continuity is achieved in her own clinic

Last week I discussed ways of providing continuity of care by using the same medical attendants. I mentioned that women coming to consultant's clinics had the opportunity to ask to see their favourite doctor or midwife and that our midwives' clinic patients are allocated to a midwife. To facilitate continuity each midwife has a different coloured sticker which is stuck to the woman's notes.

When attending St George's midwives' clinic, mothers-to-be know who they are going to see and they can carry on the conversation where they left off on their last visit. Midwives enjoy getting to know their own patients and although we have not achieved mobility of staff throughout the unit, the antenatal clinic midwives often get messages from the labour ward or the postnatal ward 'Jane Robinson is in labour, could Midwife Miranda pop up and see her please' or 'Phyllis James has had a little boy, could you tell Midwife Primo please'. So, Midwife Primo nips up to the labour ward to say hello and congratulations.

One of the most frightening aspects of labour for many women is that they will probably meet a total stranger when they enter the labour ward because, so far, most units do not operate a proper continuity scheme for maternity patients.

One way of overcoming this to some extent is for women to meet labour ward staff while they are still pregnant. At St George's, we encourage labour ward staff to come into the antenatal clinic to chat to women and introduce themselves. And when the labour ward staff are not busy they will do cardiotocographs on our pregnant women so giving them an opportunity to meet them.

In some units photographs of labour staff with names on, hang in the antenatal clinic so at least faces are recognizable.

Another feature of our clinic is the tours round the unit. At every clinic we organize a tour and many women go on the tour several times during a pregnancy. Usually our parent-craft sister takes pregnant women, their partners, their children and their friends for a tour of the labour ward to say hello to labour ward staff, to see the postnatal ward and specifically to talk to a woman who has had her baby that day so that they can see a very new baby and have an up-to-date account of labour. The tour gives women an opportunity to meet staff in the postnatal ward and the special care baby unit.

One way of achieving continuity in treatment is by using the nursing process in midwifery and in that way finding out how women feel about different aspects of their pregnancy.

At booking clinics we have a long interview with a midwife when each pregnant woman's obstetric and medical history is taken, her family's medical history, any history of abnormalities or twins noted. Her last menstrual period, whether she smokes or drinks and what sort of food she eats – in fact all the usual questions but we also add several more questions so that we can get to know each woman as an individual. For example we ask:

• What would you like us to call you?
• Have you any brothers and sisters?
• What sort of births did your mother have?
• How did she feed you all, breast or bottle?

From these questions we can find out if there is any family history of disproportion or inadequate pelvis, but even more importantly, we can find out what this women's previous conditioning to birth has been. We can discover if she was the eldest of nine and in the house when her brothers and sisters were born or that her mother only had her and it was a very difficult forceps delivery.

• Are both your parents well?
• Do they live near you?

From these questions we can discover if the mother-to-be has experienced any recent bereavements.

• Who will be able to help you when you come out of hospital with the baby?

This question will reveal how much family support the new mother believes she will receive.

We ask her about her job and whether she anticipates going back to work after the baby is born. We ask about her accommodation and whether she has enough room for a baby. All these questions give women an opportunity to think about some questions they had not thought about.

We also ask if the woman has been on the contraceptive pill and when she stopped.

• Did she mean to become pregnant at this time?
• How did she feel about the pregnancy at first?
• How did her partner react?

If the partner is present, we obviously involve him in the questions and how they both feel now. From the answers we can ascertain those women who have very ambivalent attitudes to this pregnancy and who need a lot of extra support and cherishing through pregnancy.

• Have you had anything to do with babies and little children before?

If the answer is no, an opportunity to handle a new baby while coming to the clinic can be helpful.

• Have you been in hospital before?
• How do you feel about coming here?
• Is there anything worrying you about being in hospital?

Specific requests can arise at this point and if written in the patient's notes will ensure continuity of treatment. For example, 'Joan cannot bear blood tests, she agrees to have her booking bloods taken and her 36-week blood test but she is not willing to have intermediate tests'.

• Is there anything else you would like me to write down about you?
• What about labour?
• Is there anything special you are hoping for?

The nursing process could have been made for midwifery but I will explore this subject further next week.

Reproduced with kind permission from the Nursing Mirror, December 22/29 1982.

Using the Midwifery Process

Caroline Flint explains how the nursing process can be successfully applied to midwifery and outlines how it enables antenatal care to be more satisfactory for the pregnant woman as well as giving continuity of care

One of the last questions we ask women who are booking with us is 'What about labour? Is there anything special you are hoping for?'

Some women come to the booking clinic having thought about this a great deal and can give us a very comprehensive picture of their ideal labour, but most women have not thought about labour much yet. And some women are so anxious about whether they will be able to hold on to this pregnancy because of their past history that they really cannot think so far ahead.

For those mothers-to-be who have definite ideas we can fill in their care plan for labour. For example:

'Jenny would like to avoid an episiotomy at all costs, she would prefer to avoid analgesia but if she needs something she would prefer to have a small dose of pethidine in preference to an epidural. She does not want either an enema or a perineal shave. Jenny would like the baby delivered on to her abdomen.'

'Shermaine would like to be as ambulant as possible during labour and she would like to be delivered in the birth chair.'

'Fiona would like to have an epidural as early in labour as possible. She would prefer to have an enema because she cannot bear the thought of soiling the bed. Fiona's husband Tom would very much like to cut the cord when the baby is born. Fiona would prefer not to be told the sex of the baby, she would like to look for herself.'

For most women their care plan for labour has to wait until nearer the time when they have thought about it more.

We have just introduced a 'programme for pregnancy' for each woman attending the clinic after the booking visit. This is really a diary of what the woman can expect week by week as she comes to the clinic or goes to see her GP. There is a space for her to tick off each procedure as it happens to her. There is also a space for her to put in the questions she wants to ask that day.

All women see a midwife at 28 weeks and this gives them a chance to make further additions to their care plan, to discuss breast preparation and to find out about classes.

Again at 37 weeks all women see a midwife, in the 'programme for pregnancy' it is listed in Table II.

Women keep their 'programme for pregnancy' with their co-operation card and all this can be kept safely in the Health Education Council's 'pregnancy care card'. This card is an attractive wallet for the co-operation card and it also contains questions for the women to ask herself such as 'Do I know all the benefits I can get when I'm pregnant?' and 'Have I felt my baby kick or move for the first time?'

Prospective mothers who know what to expect at each visit are strengthened by that knowledge, and by the use of these programmes. We hope to encourage women to feel that they have control over what is happening to them.

---

16 weeks – at the hospital
This week a nurse will test my urine ☐   (initial or tick) ☐
The doctor or midwife will measure my blood pressure
Check for swelling ☐   Weigh me ☐   Feel my abdomen ☐
Questions I want to ask this week ....

Table I. Care plan at 16 weeks gestation

---

37 weeks – at the hospital with a midwife

Urine test ☐	Blood pressure check ☐	Swelling ☐
Weight ☐		Abdominal palpation ☐
Discussion about labour ☐		
Questions I want to ask		

Table II. Care plan at 37 weeks gestation

Women feel that they have even more control of their pregnancy and birth if they are in control of their own notes.

At some units (St Thomas' Hospital is one) the women carry their own notes and look after them.

Notes are rarely lost and although they sometimes end up with coffee stains on them or a few scribbles this inconvenience is far less than the usual bugbear of antenatal clinic life - the lost notes.

Women take a personal interest in their own notes, they also only have one set of notes to look after. In most antenatal clinics no one has a personal interest in any of the notes and there are about 2,000 sets of records.

Notes are never static - they have either gone to the cardiac department or 'skins', or the researcher has spirited them away.

Energy and time are wasted looking for notes that have disappeared. When a woman is responsible for her own notes these problems almost disappear.

We have looked at our assessment and care plan for labour, but we are still looking at ways of using a standard care plan for the postnatal ward. To this end we are discussing with the health visitors what help they will give us with evaluating our care.

Reproduced with kind permission from Nursing Mirror, January 5 1983

Involving the Community

Volunteers helping out in the antenatal clinic can improve the atmosphere by making sure the time women spend waiting is relaxing and enjoyable. Caroline Flint outlines some of the useful tasks volunteers can undertake

Once volunteers come into an antenatal clinic the atmosphere takes on a feeling of normality and everyday life. Volunteers are ordinary people, they wear ordinary clothes, they do not look busy and rushed. They are people who have just been shopping, or who have had to wait hours for a bus, or whose children are being irritable, just normal human beings - their presence can transform the antenatal clinic.

In the third article in this series (*Nursing Mirror* December 8, 1982) I described how our creche - run by volunteers - has transformed some of our clinics. The children are happily absorbed while their mothers relax and watch our films or a demonstration, or just chat to their neighbours. The creche's benefits spill out into the everyday lives of the helpers who meet other young mothers there and so can form friendships with people in the same situation. We are fortunate in having an experienced nursery teacher to run our creche. She has wonderful ideas for the children's activities and this can be a source of learning for the women helping.

Our volunteers serve tea, coffee and soft drinks. They do not have a counter, they use an old notes trolley which has been painted. Although the trolley is rather cramped, it provides an excellent service to our waiting patients. The trolley came from the hospital store - a treasure trove of discarded furniture, old desks, filing cabinets, beds, trolleys. Whenever we need any new equipment we go and look in the store first. Every hospital has one, usually under the management of the head porter, and I recommend you investigate your hospital's store.

As often as I can, I go up to the post-natal wards to see whose new babies have arrived. As well as congratulating the mothers, I also try to recruit volunteers. Initially we ask the new mothers if they will just come and sit in the clinic and talk to the women who are waiting. In this way the mothers can talk about their stay in St George's, how their labour went, what it is like now they have a baby, how the brothers and sisters are coping, and the sleepless nights. In short, they describe how they manage and what they find difficult.

We make a date with the new mother for when the baby is about two months old. On the letter of invitation we encourage her to feed the baby in the clinic - only if she would like to, of course - change the baby's nappy, bath the baby. In fact we ask her to do as little or as much as she feels able.

This 'live teaching aid' creates great interest. Many women hold a splendid session without any prompting, but some women are shy and need the occasional help. We prompt them by asking 'Was there anything confusing about life in the postnatal ward? What about your stitches? How soon did you feel comfortable again? Have you told them about your labour? Can you tell Cathy here about epidurals, she is thinking of having one.'

A baby being bathed in the clinic is a beautiful sight especially once the baby has got to the smiling, cooing stage and enjoys a lovely splashy bath. In some areas there are local voluntary organizations which can put on this sort of interest session, for example the National Childbirth Trust, the Twins Club, the La Leche League or the Association of Breast-Feeding Mothers.

One of our newer ventures is a 'nearly new' baby clothes stall - we do not charge more than ten pence for most articles. This is proving enormously popular with both mothers-to-be and helpers. We hope to go on to maternity clothes - either to be hired or to be sold cheaply - the funds to go to the League of Friends to benefit the antenatal clinic. It is amazing how the pennies mount up, and it gives everyone a great boost when they can look at a specific piece of equipment, or at a special treat - such as a piece of cake for everyone coming to the clinic on a special occasion - and they can say 'We raised the money to do that'.

At the West London Hospital there is a monthly bra-fitting evening when women who are interested in buying a maternity bra can come and be properly fitted. This gives an opportunity for women to chat to each other and to discuss breastfeeding and pregnancy with other women.

Recently at the South London Hospital for Women, an evening panel discussion was held. On the panel was a consultant obstetrician, a midwifery nursing officer, a community health council member and a journalist. The audience was able to ask questions, discuss, challenge and provoke thought - it was a venture worth repeating.

In the antenatal clinic will be women and men with many varied talents - it is worth tapping them. What about a singer performing in the middle of the occasional clinic, or a violinist? What about an evening play? *Holding the Baby* by Rony Robinson immediately comes to mind - it is a brilliant play about a couple expecting their first baby, it needs no scenery and has only two characters.

Everyone attending the clinic can be asked to bring their old magazines and to look out for articles of interest for the midwives. One of our most successful ventures has been our 'for sale' board; admittedly it does attract the weirdest of items for sale - among the prams and nearly-new maternity clothes nestles a coach tour to Rimini, several cars and a furnished flat complete with 'dinning room' (*sic*).

Our plans for the future include an antenatal 'get-to-know-you-scheme'. We are looking for a volunteer with local knowledge who can match up people who live near each other- perhaps with the aid of a large wall map and coloured pins.

In the next few weeks the postnatal ward sister and I will be starting postnatal groups in the antenatal clinic. These are basically support groups where people can come and talk to other people going through the same experiences. I have led these before and have found it often helps to hang the discussion round a specific topic, for example: sex after the baby's birth; the things I miss most from before I had the baby; and can you cope on one income?

As long as everyone feels free to bring up any topic they wish to discuss, the original subject always gets buried under what is actually troubling people at the time. Perhaps from our group exciting things may grow - such as a postnatal support system. The possibilities are endless.

Reproduced with kind permission from Nursing Mirror, January 12 1983.

Growing in Confidence

Caroline Flint explains how the midwives who work at her clinic have gained in confidence because they have been involved in improvements to the antenatal service

Midwives who choose to work in an antenatal clinic usually do so for a variety of reasons. Many midwives have small children or family commitments and work part-time. Some of the midwives are not physically strong enough to cope with the lifting that has to be done on the labour ward or postnatal ward. Some have been inspired and interested by the challenge pregnant women bring them, others are there because they 'have been sent': Because part-time staff arrive on duty at different times and because, unlike working in a ward, there is no report when all the staff gather together a special effort has to be made to encourage antenatal clinic staff to relate to each other and form a cohesive team.

In our clinic we have a weekly 'working lunch'. We all bring sandwiches and discuss and explore different topics together. Sometimes we see a film or a video, or preview one of the visual aids for the clinic. On other occasions we discuss ways of improving the service we are providing. Each member of the team has a different point of view and we try to encourage everyone to participate. The student nurses see things that some of us, who have been around for a long time, stopped seeing years ago. Sometimes we try to analyse why a particular clinic went so well, and sometimes why a particular clinic went so badly.

We tried role play when we first brought in the assessment for the nursing process and we plan to use it again. It is such a useful educational tool and it is such fun to do.

We air grievances and try to smooth out hitches, we allocate or volunteer for specific jobs. One of the most useful ventures is when we visit another antenatal clinic to see how they organise themselves - this has many benefits.

It means that we all, or a group of us, go out together; this is refreshing and enjoyable and helps us all to get to know each other better. Seeing another clinic functioning opens our eyes to different ways of approaching antenatal care. Some of the ideas we can utilize, others we regretfully discard. One great benefit we gain from these outings is that we appreciate the benefits we have, for example we have remarked 'I wouldn't like to work with that consultant, would you? I've never met anyone so grumpy. Thank goodness for our lovely ones.'

'Have you ever seen anything as poky as those consulting rooms, ours are so much better.'

'I'd hate to be a midwife there, they don't do anything except weigh patients.'

We all work together keeping statistics for our clinic - this involves no more than a tatty piece of paper outside each consulting room on which we jot down how many patients were seen by each person. These figures are helpful for the sister/hostess allocating women to different medical attendants and they encourage us when we find that last week, out of a total of 296 follow-on patients seen, 113 were seen by midwives, or the week before - when a total of 283 follow-on patients were seen in our clinic - 70 of them by midwives.

We try to use each team member's special skills: one midwife is quiet and reliable, she does all the ordering of pharmacy and stocks; one midwife is an early bird and she prepares the clinics; one is more mechanical than most, she threads the projector; and one is very tidy, she keeps an eye on the posters and leaflets which tend to straggle.

Our auxiliary nurse has a great clerical aptitude, she is also a very warm and welcoming person - she looks after all the clerical work attached to the booking clinic and welcomes new patients. Some of the midwives see their role as hostesses to frightened, nervous mothers-to-be. The midwives give welcoming talks to women when they first arrive, or go round and talk to women waiting in the clinic, or they stand in for sister on a Friday when there is 'open house' for anyone who has a worry or problem to come and discuss it over a cup of coffee. Some midwives love seeing pregnant women for the complete consultation and some prefer to chaperone doctors.

As our midwives' clinic progresses, so the confidence of the midwives who run it, grows. Seeing the same women month by month, and then week by week, shows the midwife that she is perfectly capable of giving antenatal care. And this makes her more alert to signs that all is not going well because she knows the women so well. Her confidence is increased by the attitude of the women she sees - they respect and trust her, and they look forward to seeing her. As the doctors see the quality of care their patients receive they become happier with the midwives' clinic and more aware of its benefits, to the women, to the midwives, to the doctors.

Our next step at either midwives' or consultants' clinics will be to discuss cases as they crop up, after the clinic. This is done at Sighthill Health Centre. 'At the end of each clinic all members of the [community] team gather to review management decisions. Each member who has seen patients relates risk factors which have arisen and decisions which have been taken.'

More than ever, this will help us all to feel like a team and will make us more responsive and sensitive to the women.

Thank you for all your letters - next week I shall be quoting from many of them with some really interesting ideas on improving our service.

Reproduced with kind permission from Nursing Mirror, January 19 1983

Encouraging Feedback

Caroline Flint was overwhelmed by the response to this series, which looked at ways of improving antenatal care for mothers-to-be, midwives and consultants. The comments were varied: some critical; some enthusiastic; but all were constructive

It was rewarding to receive so many letters and phone calls in response to this series. My overwhelming impression is that antenatal clinic staff nationwide are trying out new ideas in order to make their clinics more attractive to mothers. Everywhere midwives are talking about how to change, how to streamline, how to 'humanize' their service. Many of the letters were from women who had recently experienced the 'system' and were extremely happy with the efforts being made on their behalf. Several women mentioned specific hospitals, midwives and consultants by name.

Shared care with GPs was extremely popular and several women mentioned with pleasure the care they had received from their doctors and community midwives. They felt that they could talk with the GPs or midwives for as long as they needed, and that the GPs and midwives were interested in them as a person.

In an interesting letter from Heavitrees Hospital in Exeter I read about a proposal that booking histories may be taken in the privacy of a women's own home by the community midwife. I think this is a lovely humane idea. In conjunction with this are plans for the further integration of hospital and community midwives. Surely the next step from this idea is that the community midwife attends the clinic when the client she had booked in comes for her first visit.

From the letters it was apparent that community midwives help at several hospital antenatal clinics, but sadly it seemed that this happened when the community midwives had not many community clinics.

Midwifery management was mentioned and how important it is, if changes are to be made, that managers should be supportive and encouraging. It was also said how much easier it is to effect change with support from 'above', I know how much this has helped us at St George's.

Not only does the manager's attitude matter enormously; so does the consultant obstetrician's attitude. Some consultants can be very involved and encouraging. At St George's we are fortunate to have consultants who are willing to come to a monthly meeting with me to discuss ways to improve the antenatal clinic. With this support we have been able to increase the midwife involvement and to try many different ideas.

Sadly, some obstetricians feel the need to monopolise the patients which leads to the situation I saw recently. I met a consultant obstetrician who reckoned that out of a clinic containing 100 patients he had to see at least 50 of them. I pointed out that the clinic only lasted three hours, which meant that on average he was spending under four minutes with each women, not counting him answering the phone, stopping for a cup of tea, talking with colleagues.

As the National Childbirth Trust's report *Change in Antenatal Care* says: 'It is not surprising that women feel disappointed when they are in and out of the examination room in a matter of minutes and have no opportunity for discussion or for voicing anxieties.'

Another paragraph from *Change in Antenatal Care* says: 'The convergence of 100 or more expectant mothers on an overcrowded antenatal clinic within a period of two hours is bound to produce stress however well organized the clinic and well intentioned each single member of staff. It is an unsatisfactory experience for all concerned, in some ways as much for the doctors, nurses, midwives and clerks working in the clinic as it is for the women required to attend it. Women feel that they are on a conveyor belt which must be kept moving at all costs; doctors are under intolerable pressure to keep the flow through, and feel guilty because under such circumstances it is impossible to give adequate care; and midwives, deprived of the opportunity to exercise their professional skills, experience dissatisfaction and frustration in their role.'

I received some suggestions that consultant obstetricians might find great satisfaction in being 'real' consultants, that is that their role might become peripatetic, looking in on midwives and doctors seeing patients, or to be available for referrals or lead a 'teaching round' on the different rooms in the antenatal clinic.

I received some exciting ideas from the nursing officer and sisters of Queen Charlotte's antenatal clinic. They have files containing articles of interest for the patients to read and they encourage the women to bring in articles for inclusion in their library.

At Queen Charlotte's they are also thinking of having a 'suggestions box' for patients to put ideas into and they are making a video about what their hospital offers from pregnancy right through to the postnatal ward. This tape will then be shown at evening sessions.

A few weeks ago, a student nurse came to our clinic and criticized our booking clinics as being far too clinical. He suggested that we should invite a group of women and their partners to see a film about antenatal care, introduce them to each other, and that a midwife should take their histories then. He felt that the emphasis would be of a social nature rather than a medical one at that session.

Stress the social side

This feeling also has come through when I have talked with others involved with delivering antenatal care - that is, our emphasis is on the medical aspects of pregnancy. For the mothers-to-be it would be much better to stress the more social and emotional aspects with the need to take blood pressures and palpate abdomens still there but not the main reason for coming.

At Queen Charlotte's, the staff also have plans for on-going evaluation by both staff and clients, demonstrations in the waiting area, evening booking appointments with plenty of time being allocated to each women, discussion groups for postnatal parents and a book list for prospective parents.

Many letters stressed the enormous value of having somewhere where the children could play. At Heavitrees Hospital they use volunteer helpers and at King's they use nursery nurses.

In a letter from King's College Hospital, and in several other letters, midwife allocation is described. At the booking clinic each midwife is allocated an equal number of patients. She then puts a sticker on the front of the notes with her name on. Each time the woman attends the antenatal clinic, the same midwife sees her and only refers her to a doctor when necessary. Many hospitals have specific times when women see the consultant - we always send women at 36 weeks to see the consultant, and earlier if the baby is presenting by the breech.

Other suggestions included a 'problems room' where a senior midwife sits throughout the clinic so that she is available to answer questions that have not been answered during their consultations. Another idea is to place a midwife at the exit of the clinic saying goodbye to women as they leave and asking 'Everything all right?' or 'Are you happy about everything?' In this way, the women are encouraged to voice any queries or worries they have.

Some clinics have an open invitation to women to come and have a 'cuppa' with sister to talk about their worries, or questions they have about what goes on at that particular hospital. Women are more likely to come if there is a specific time each week when a sister is available. I have found that women who are not even booked at St George's will come to have a cup of coffee with me on a Friday at 11.00h. This can cause some embarrassment when one's opinion is asked on treatment being given at other hospitals, but relieves quite a bit of anxiety in women who want to compare what each hospital in the area has to offer.

I picked up a useful tip on a visit to King's College Hospital. This was to have a selection of commonly prescribed drugs on hand in the antenatal clinic, so that our patients do not have to queue for ages in the pharmacy. We have a selection of different iron preparations, treatments for thrush, simple antibiotics, antacids and folic acid tablets. This cuts down the total length of the visit for women needing extra drugs, rather than just our usual iron tablets.

The student nurse who was unhappy about our booking clinic, was also concerned about how little we involve fathers. This needs considerable thought, because he was right in his observation that, despite the fact that husbands are always welcomed to our clinics and, indeed, often come, husbands are still somehow left sitting there like a 'spare part'. We need to ask them and their wives how we can involve them more.

Some letters emphasized the poor communication between hospital and GP: blood results and culture results taking two to three weeks to arrive at the doctor's; ultrasound results not being notified to the GP or haemoglobin results at 28 weeks. Much appreciation was expressed for the letter of welcome we send to all our pregnant women before the booking clinic.

I was fascinated by the large number of women who have small children and are working in the health service. I was gratified that they were able to make time to read *Nursing Mirror* and write to me. I was over-whelmed with admiration for these women, remembering how demanding it was bringing up tiny children. But it also made me realize that there is a huge untapped source of knowledge and experience about working mothers in the NHS. It also made me wonder if I was supporting working mothers on my staff enough. How many hospitals run nurseries for their shift workers? How many have a list of registered child minders in the immediate vicinity?

Since I started to write this series, two reports have come out that are worth reading. *Maternity Care in Action*, the first report of the Maternity Services Advisory Committee, has checklists for helping clinic staff to review what they need to do; this costs 55 pence and is available from HMSO. And the *Report of the RCOG Working Party on Antenatal and Intrapartum Care*, which is available from the Royal College of Obstetricians and Gynaecologists, 27 Sussex Place, London NW1 4RG.

Thanks go to all those readers who sent me their comments and suggestions. To Mrs Murray, director of maternity services, Mrs Afari and Miss Rawana, nursing officers, Professor Chamberlain, Mr Amias and Mrs Varma, consultant obstetricians. To the staff midwives, staff nurse and auxiliary nurse with whom I work in the clinic. To the staff in the labour, antenatal and postnatal wards and to our clerical staff and volunteers.

References

Boddy, K., Parboosingh, J., Shepherd, C. *A Schematic Approach to Prenatal Care.* Department of Obstetrics and Gynaecology, Edinburgh University.

Boyd, C., Sellers, L. (1982). *The British Way of Birth.* Pan Books.

Chamberlain, G. (1978). 'A re-examination of antenatal care.' *Journal of the Royal Society of Medicine*, 71, September.

Chng, P., MacGillivray, I. (1980). 'An audit of antenatal care: The value of the first antenatal visit.' *British Medical Journal*, 281, November 1.

DHSS (1980). *Perinatal and Neonatal Mortality.* Second report from the Social Services Committee. HMSO.

Hall, M., Chng, P., MacGillivray, I. (1980). 'Is routine antenatal care worthwhile?' *The Lancet,* July 12.

Kitzinger, S. (1978). *Women as Mothers.* Fontana Books.

MacIntyre, S. (1980). 'Interaction in antenatal clinics.' Paper given at Research and the Midwife conference, Glasgow.

National Childbirth Trust (1981). *Change in Antenatal Care.* Report from working party set up for the NCT by Sheila Kitzinger.

Oakley, A. (1979). *From Here to Maternity. Becoming a Mother.* Penguin Books.

Oakley, A. (1980). *Women Confined. Towards a Sociology of Childbirth.* Martin Robertson and Co. Ltd.

Spastics Society (1981). *Who's Holding the Baby Now?*

Spastics Society. *Feeling Special.* A film about care before birth, produced by Randel Evans Productions Ltd, directed by Nigel Evans.

Reproduced with kind permission from Nursing Mirror, January 26 1983

Do Antenatal Clinics have to be Cattle markets?

This article discusses what hospital midwives can do to improve their own clinics tomorrow, or next week, simple thoughts and ideas which wouldn't take months of consultation with obstetricians, nursing officers, policy making committees and procedure meetings

Having spent considerable effort and time persuading expectant mothers to crowd into centralized antenatal clinics in consultant obstetric units we are now faced with the task of trying to make these clinics less like cattle markets - less overcrowded, less noisy, less unpleasant. And to do this we need to reverse the whole process again by making them smaller, quieter, more personal, more intimate.

In this article I wish to set aside the whole philosophy of whether pregnant women have any place inside a hospital at all, unless they are diabetic or have serious cardiac conditions, and the fact that for most women it is much easier, therefore less stressful, to go to a health centre near their home. Midwives need to make their voices heard and need to be pushing for clinics in the community run by community midwives and GPs, and for home antenatal visits by community midwives.

How can we make our own clinics smaller, more intimate? How can we change things easily and simply? Firstly we need to work out when women in our own clinics are seen by a midwife and this may work out something like this - women having shared care with their GP and community midwife will be seen in the community at 16, 20, 24, 30, 32, 34, 37, 39 weeks, and maybe at the hospital at 12, 28, 36, 38 and 40 weeks. At 12 weeks they will have their history taken by a midwife and will then be examined by

an obstetrician, in many hospitals the woman will have her 28 week consultation with the midwives because they can then give her the Certificate of Expected Confinement, and can arrange her parentcraft classes; she would therefore only see an obstetrician if the midwife was concerned about anything. The 36 week visit would be with a consultant obstetrician and the 40 week visit with a senior registrar, but many obstetricians are happy for the 38 week visit to be with the midwives so that the woman can discuss her final plans and wishes for labour, and can have a long discussion about the forthcoming labour with the midwife. Thus a woman going through the system of shared care like this, could expect to see a hospital midwife at 12 weeks, 28 weeks and 38 weeks. With the present system it is highly likely that the pregnant woman would meet different midwives at each of these appointments but this can be transformed if each midwife carries a diary with times when she can be consulted, i.e. her own appointment system, this does not necessarily have to be at the time of a consultant's clinic, it could even be at a time when she can find spare room with a couch, because in a consultant obstetric unit, if a doctor is required there are always several available on a bleep, and anyway the number of women needing medical referral will be very small.

Let us take Mrs Rhoda Phipps as an example - she is a primigravida who is having shared care with her GP and she comes to the hospital with her GP letter at 12 weeks where she meets Midwife Brown at the booking clinic who takes her history. When Midwife Brown has taken her history Rhoda will be examined by a doctor but before this she makes an appointment in her diary for February 14th when Rhoda will be 28 weeks pregnant and for 27th April when she will be 38 weeks pregnant. She writes these appointments on Rhoda's appointment card and also writes her name Midwife Lorna Brown on Rhoda's appointment card so that Rhoda knows who is 'her' midwife at the hospital, if ever Rhoda needs to telephone the hospital she can ask to speak to 'her' midwife and when Mrs Phipps has seen a doctor she can seek out Midwife Lorna Brown to explain anything she doesn't understand and to make clear anything that has confused or upset her. When Mrs Phipps is in labour she can send a message to the antenatal clinic so that her midwife can pop up and see her.

With women who are not having shared care with their GPs far more of the visits a pregnant woman makes to the hospital can be with a midwife, with low risk women the Royal College of Obstetricians in their Report of a Working Party on Antenatal and Intrapartum Care[1] suggest that a woman should see an obstetrician at 12, 30 and 40 weeks and at other times (16, 22, 26, 34, 36 and 38 weeks) should be seen by a midwife or GP. If individual midwives carry a diary and make themselves responsible for a group of women - taking on each week as many as they can manage - several benefits accrue: the woman sees the same midwife throughout her pregnancy, the midwife has the pleasure of seeing an individual woman through pregnancy. The woman taken out of the system in this way could reduce the numbers crowding into consultants' clinics and so enable them to be less stressful and more efficient. Similarly, if a woman does not turn up for a Clinic she is far more likely to phone and explain, if she knows that she will actually be missed by someone who is interested in her progress. If you are thinking how much you should like to take on responsibility for a number of pregnant women but your clinic is short of room, remember that for an antenatal consultation all you need is a space with a couch or bed in it and preferably two chairs so that you and your patient can sit and talk to each other. The ideal - a consulting room with couch, desk and 2 chairs, the almost ideal - someone's office with a couch in it (ask your head porter if he has any spare couches), the fairly ideal - a labour ward with a delivery bed and two chairs in it and the not quite so ideal - a bed curtained off in the postnatal ward.

Most midwives can find a small space that they can use for 'just this morning' or 'just this afternoon' and in every hospital there are offices that are unused for periods, perhaps every Wednesday afternoon or for two hours on a Friday morning.

When obstetricians are approached by midwives wishing to make the provision of antenatal care to women more humane and pleasant they are invariably very supportive and enthusiastic and only too happy to go along with the RCOG Document[1]. This is an opportunity for hospital midwives to practice fully as midwives and to gain and receive a great deal of pleasure both from and for the women they are caring for.

Reference

1. Royal College of Obstetricians and Gynaecologists (1982). *Report of the R.C.O.G. Working Party on Antenatal and Intrapartum Care.* September.

Reproduced with kind permission from Midwife, Health Visitor and Community Nurse, Vol. 20, October 1984

An Antenatal Adventure

What happens when a young girl finds she's pregnant? Caroline Flint imagines her ideal progress and suggests the kind of support she needs, and should find, at her local clinic

I'm going to take part in a celebration, I'm starting on a journey which will change my life. At the end of this journey I will be a different woman; society's concept of me will be different and my concept of myself will be different. Nothing will ever be the same again. I am embarking on the greatest adventure of my life - I think I'm pregnant.

I've been feeling sick in the mornings for the past week, my breasts are tingling and uncomfortable and I'm two weeks late with my period. Today I'm going to the pregnancy clinic. I know where to go because it's advertised in the local newsagents, the chemist's and in the local 'freebie' newspaper. You know the sort of advert: 'Think you might be pregnant? Why not pop along and talk to one of our midwives - Tuesday and Thursday evenings from 6-9 pm'.

I go into the hospital and there are clear directions with pictures of pregnant women and arrows pointing towards where I have to go. When I get to the clinic, which the arrows have led me to, it is a big room with a desk and two ladies sitting at it. On the desk are two big notices 'Midwife Julie' and 'Midwife Merle'. I go to the desk feeling very embarrassed and shy and midwife Julie looks up from what she is writing. She smiles and me and says: 'Hello, can I help you?' And then I say the words that will change my life ' 'I think I might be pregnant'.

'Well, let's go and see' says Julie and we go off together to do a pregnancy test. She tells me that the test is positive and asks me how I feel about the news.

Now that it's definite, I feel a bit shocked. Julie and I have a cup of tea together and she gently asks me about myself. Like what sort of things I'm eating, whether I smoke or drink or take any drugs, how I'm placed financially, whether my boyfriend is around and about my family. She takes my blood pressure because, she says, she likes to get an initial reading and she weighs me. While we are talking she jots down details on a set of case notes.

When we've finished chatting and I'm feeling ready to go, Julie introduces me to Merle who is her partner. She then asks me if I will come and see her again in four weeks' time and she gives me a date and time which is convenient for me. If I wanted a termination I know she would refer me to a gynaecologist at this stage. She then hands me my case notes and asks me to bring them with me whenever I come. But, she says, if I want her to, she will keep them for me. Because I'm not sure how my news will be received at home, I ask her to keep the case notes for the time being.

But I never turned up for my next appointment. When I told Gary about the baby he went off in a huff, and my dad threatened to throw me out. I've never felt so miserable in my life. Two days later I got a letter from Julie and Merle saying that they hoped I was all right and that they'd been looking forward to seeing me again.

Of course, I went after that. It was so nice to see a friendly, familiar face and I told Julie all about the problems I was having. I cried and we had a cup of tea together. She then wrote down more details about me, such as how my mother had all her babies, whether we had been breastfed or not, how close I was to my family, where I was living and how much room I had, what illnesses I'd had in the past and whether I'd had any operations or accidents or blood transfusions.

This time she took some blood from me and again took my blood pressure, weighed me and tested my urine. She also felt my tummy to see if she could feel anything yet. She couldn't, but she asked me to keep a note of when the baby began to move. She asked me how I was eating and we discussed the sort of diet I should be aiming for - fewer chips and more oranges and protein every day.

After that visit I took my case notes home with me. My mum was really interested in everything Julie had written down and, in the end, so was my dad. They decided to come with me the next time I went to see Julie. But, by then, as it turned out, Gary had come back again. He had just felt so overwhelmed at the thought of having a baby on the way.

I saw my friends Julie and Merle throughout my pregnancy, except when I went to see the obstetrician at 16 and 36 weeks. Though they didn't deliver my baby, Merle came to see me when I was in labour (it was a Saturday). And one of them popped in to see me every day on the postnatal ward, except for Sundays when they were both off duty.

Later I found out that Merle and Julie worked part-time — they both did 20 hours a week. Julie worked all day on Mondays and Fridays in the antenatal clinic having antenatal consultations (she did seven hours on those days) and Merle did the same on Wednesdays and Saturdays.

Merle and Julie each worked three hours together on Tuesday and Thursday evenings for women to 'drop in' to their booking clinic. Between them they saw 200 follow-on patients a month and about 50 new 'bookers' a month. They were hospital-based midwives but they could just as easily have been community midwife Julie working with GP Merle, or community midwives Merle and Julie working with GP Flora. At my hospital there were also two other midwives who worked in partnership. Jane and Masie did Monday and Wednesday evenings and two full days a week each.

Working in this way four part-time midwives could provide full antenatal care for nearly 500 women a year (except for the two consultant visits). They provide continuity by popping into the labour ward and postnatal ward and they also provide an excellent booking and referral service during the evenings. This could provide a cheap, pleasant and caring service. It is not as comprehensive as a team providing full continuity of care, but better than the care many women receive at present.

Further reading
Report of the RCOG Working Party on Antenatal and Intrapartum Care £1 from the RCOG at 27 Sussex Place, Regent's Park, London NW1 4RG

Reproduced with kind permission from Nursing Times, January 23, 1985

Labour of Love

Exciting things are happening in midwifery in South London. Some mothers at St George's are able to opt for total midwifery care from booking clinic to post-discharge follow-up in a 'know your midwife' scheme. Over the next few weeks, the midwives involved, the researcher and some of the mothers describe what it is like to be part of the scheme. Here Caroline Flint, the scheme's prime mover, explains how the system works

At St George's Hospital, Tooting, we are evolving a new breed of midwife, neither a community midwife nor a hospital midwife, but a midwife who is equally at home in both environments. I think that this is the midwife of the future; someone who uses the best of both environments for the comfort, happiness and safety of pregnant women.

A woman who comes to the normal booking clinic at St George's has a medical and social history taken and she is examined by a doctor. A further appointment is made for her next consultation.

After each booking clinic, I go through all the notes, discarding those where women are having shared care with their GP and those women who would obviously be classed as high risk. Then, one of the senior registrars and I agree whether these women are suitable for almost total midwife care, Our criteria are:
- Over 5ft in height
- No previous uterine surgery
- No previous intra-uterine growth retardation
- No previous stillbirths or neonatal deaths
- No more than a total of two terminations or miscarriages
- No gross medical conditions

The notes of mothers designated as suitable for midwife care are stamped and then left for our research assistant who pins envelopes on them. Inside half the envelopes is a piece of paper which says ' know your midwife scheme' and in the other half is a piece of paper which says 'control group.'

The women who have been randomized into the know your midwife group then receive a letter from us which details the scheme. It tells them that if they want to come on the scheme they will be looked after by this group of four midwives throughout their pregnancy (except when they see their consultant obstetrician at 36 weeks). When they go into labour they will be looked after by one of the midwives, and after they have had their baby they will be visited by the midwives from the team. When they go home the midwives from the team will look after them there. They are sent a new appointment for the know your midwife antenatal clinic.

This service is offered to 20 women a month. Most of them return our tear-off slip accepting the scheme. A few women do not want to be looked after by midwives only – they prefer more medical care – but the vast majority are eager to join us. (Actual numbers will be given when our research is published in a year's time.)

Throughout her pregnancy the woman (and often her partner) will come for antenatal consultations with the four midwives. We hold clinics every afternoon and on Wednesday evenings until 9pm. On Friday afternoons we do not usually hold a clinic but do antenatal consultations in the women's houses. We discuss the woman's choices about when she will leave hospital after the baby is born, and what she should get ready for her home-coming.

When the woman goes into labour she rings the hospital and asks the switchboard to bleep the know your midwife on call. Whoever is on call rings the woman back and discusses when she should come into hospital. If the woman sounds as if she is in very early labour, the midwife will sometimes go to her home to assess whether she is in established labour or not. Women find this immensely reassuring. (Discontinued, October 1984).

If the midwife and the woman have decided that it is to early for her to go into hospital they keep in touch on the telephone. They usually arrange a time when they can meet at the hospital. The on-call scheme midwives are not necessarily in hospital; they have long-range bleeps which give them a great deal of freedom, and may be at home or out shopping.

The scheme midwife tries to reach the hospital before the woman so that she can arrange a room and prepare the notes ready for the reception of the mother-to-be and her partner, or partners and friends.

While the woman is in labour, her midwife is with her. The scheme midwives refer straight to the registrar on duty in the labour ward and, for most of their cases, work with just a medical or midwifery student. The student midwives who are in their free allocation period at the end of their training are also beginning to work with the team. Otherwise, the team looks out for any students who happen to be allocated to the labour ward. The women are usually happy to have a student with them as long as one of the midwives they know conducts the delivery.

The scheme midwife conducts the delivery, or if the woman has a forceps delivery she assists with that. She then transfers the mother and baby to the postnatal ward when they are ready to go. During the woman's stay there, one of the team visits in the mornings, and the midwife on call (unless she is in the middle of a delivery) calls again in the evening. On discharge, the team visits the mother and baby daily if they live within the Wandsworth health district. They are visited daily until the tenth day, then about every four-seven days up to 28 days, as appropriate.

As a midwife, working this way is delightful. It gives us great joy to be able to be with a group of women all the way through their pregnancy, labour and puerperium and experience is gained quickly and easily because of the continuity of care we are able to give. If a woman develops complications we can still go on caring for her because we are hospital-based, and she has a midwife with her anyway. Thus, we can scrub for her Caesarean section, attend her during her trial of labour, and top up her epidural.

The system breaks down at times. In 15 months we have had four occasions when we have had more than one woman in the labour ward. We have then had to rely on labour ward staff to help us out. They are very willing to do this, because as they say: ' They are all hospital patients and it's so nice to have an extra pair of hands when a scheme midwife comes in with a woman.'

One of the staff midwives in the labour ward keeps a count of our statistics for us, and we have been touched by the welcoming attitude of most of the staff.

In the postnatal ward we rely on the regular staff a great deal as we attend to our women in the mornings and evenings only. They have indeed been marvellous, treating us as a bonus. After the regular staff have been allocated a number of women for the day, they say that it is helpful when a scheme midwife comes in and offers: 'Don't worry about Mrs ..., I'll look after her.' The research findings will be important for midwives every where because they will show whether it is safe to let midwives look after low- risk women almost entirely. The midwives we work with appreciate this and we have been overwhelmed by their support.

It is not all hunky-dory of course. There are times when we are very tired – about every six weeks we work a very long span of duty. Midwives who have not experienced bearing the full responsibility for their practice before, sometimes find it can be very heavy.

One of the loveliest aspects of working in a small team is the support we all gain from each other. A real bond of affection has grown up between us; we try and help each other out when someone is tired, or if someone's child has an event at school. We feel relaxed with each other and we are able to be open with each other without feeling threatened, knowing that the other person will understand. Weekly meetings are an essential part of the scheme. We hold them on Wednesday afternoons when we have a break of two hours in the antenatal clinic.

The scheme midwives do one of two spans of duty. On early shift (E) the midwife comes on duty at 8.00am, nursing the postnatal women in the postnatal ward on the scheme. She then goes into the community to nurse women there, returning at lunchtime and for an antenatal clinic in the afternoon (for five or six women), except at weekends when she has a half day. On call (OC), the midwife is in call from 7.45 am one day until 7.45 am the following day. She comes into the hospital only for labouring women, except from 6.00pm – 9.00pm when she nurses the scheme women who are in the postnatal ward.

On Wednesdays there is another span of duty from 1.00 – 9.00pm, when the midwife spends all that time in the antenatal clinic seeing scheme women, except from 4.00 – 6.00pm when she and the others are having a meeting.

The midwives tot up their hours of duty each month. They should do 150 hours every 28 days. If they have done too many these are adjusted every few months and they have extra days off, of if they have done too few hours (rare) we just wait and they catch up. The present off-duty is shown in Fig 1.

This scheme seems to give women the continuity they have been wanting so much for so long. For midwives, the scheme allows them to know their off-duty months in advance, and it gives them the joy of being able to look after women in a very satisfying way. At the moment, the rota can be demanding and it seems to me that in the future it will beneficial to have teams of six midwives who will be able to look after 300-350 women a year. Because the team is bigger there will have to be more effort in helping the women to meet all the midwives, and with this aim in mind, in the rota I have included tea parties and coffee mornings (Fig 2). I have also included times for antenatal classes given by the team. Like the previous rota for four midwives (which has only three lines), the specimen rota has only five lines even though it is for six midwives. This is because the six midwives will have 42 weeks' holiday between them and study periods, and the sixth midwife fits in there (she is marked as * on the rota).

In this rota, on-call is from midnight-to-midnight. The early shift is as before, there is late duty of 1.00-9.00pm and I envisage the midwives on this shift working in the postnatal ward or in the clinic when there is an evening session. We now have our evening clinics on Wednesdays and these would fit in on that day. If two teams were to work in this way and the rota was staggered so that when one team was on week 1, the other team was on week 2, the postnatal ward would be covered by a know your midwife all the time except for Friday and Saturday evenings and night duty. This would make the teams much more self-sufficient than at present; 12 midwives could look after 600-700 women a year plus the midwives needed to staff the postnatal ward at night and the part-time midwife working Friday and Saturday evenings. One of the most important parts of the scheme would still be the regular weekly meeting for all the midwives – a source of great comfort and strength.

Mon	Tues	Wed	Thur	Fri	Sat	Sun	Mon	Tues	Wed	Thur	Fri	Sat	Sun	Mon
DO	DO	OC	E	OC	1/2	OC	E	OC	E	DO	DO	OC	1/2	OC
E	OC	E	DO	DO	OC	1/2	OC	E	1-9	OC	E	DO	DO	DO
OC	E	1-9	OC	E	DO	DO	DO	DO	OC	E	OC	1/2	OC	E
*		*		*		*		*		*		*		*

Tue	Wed	Thur	Fri	Sat	Sun	
E	1-9	OC	E	DO	DO	The rota repeats itself every three weeks — the fourth
DO	OC	E	OC	1/2	OC	midwife (*) fills in for holidays and time owed
OC	E	DO	DO	OC	1/2	
*	*	*	*	*	*	

Fig. 1 Current off-duty

Sun	Mon	Tue	Wed	Thu	Fri	Sat	Sun	Mon	Tue	Wed	Thu	Fri	Sat	Sun
1-9	E	DO	E	OC	E	DO	DO	DO	E	E	OC	E	OC	1-9
E	OC	1-9	E	E	DO	DO	DO	E	OC	1-9	E	DO	E	E
DO	DO	E	OC	1-9	E	OC	E	OC	1-9	E	DO	E	DO	DO
DO	E	OC	1-9	E	OC	E	OC	E	DO	1-9	E	DO	DO	DO
OC	1-9	DO	1-9	E	DO	DO	DO	1-9	E	OC	E	OC	E	OC
*	*	*	*	*	*	*	*	*	i	*	*	*	*	*

	c			m				c	c	m	c			
	l			e				l	o	e	o			
	a			e				a	f	e	f			
	s			t				s	f	t	f			
	s			i				s	e	i	e			
				n					e	n	e			
				g						g				

The rota repeats itself every two weeks.

Fig. 2 Specimen rota

Because we have been given freedom to develop, we have been able to respond to the needs of the women we serve and to our needs as midwives, as mothers and members of our families or social environments. The person who has given us the freedom to develop is the same person who has financed the scheme and who has found us office space and equipment, our director of midwifery services.

The other people who deserve our thanks are the midwives, enrolled nurses and nursery nurses in the rest of the unit. We may see ourselves as the midwives of the future, but at the moment we are an anomaly which does not always fit in with the normal functioning of the unit. But, because of the generosity of our colleagues, the women are looked after to the best of everyone's ability, and a great many of them write to extol the scheme and to commiserate with their less fortunate sisters who have to have their babies 'the ordinary way'.

Reproduced with kind permission from Nursing Times, January 30 1985.

Bedside Manners

Midwives should be aware of climbing the hierarchy and losing their skills at the bedside. Caroline Flint argues for a radical rethink of how the profession should be organized

When we midwives separate ourselves from women we do ourselves harm - after all the term midwife means 'with woman'. I'm thinking about the management of our profession and the damage we have done to ourselves by adopting the hierarchy of nursing - and in so doing we have separated ourselves from our reason for existing: pregnant women and their babies.

At the moment midwives are led, administered or 'managed' by people with such ambiguous titles as chief nursing officer, district nursing officer, director of nursing studies (midwifery), nursing officer, special projects officer or sister. Some units, aware of the loss of identity of the midwife which is present in these titles, are now appointing senior midwives instead of nursing officers or even midwifery specialists, but as far as I can see the change in title does not necessarily go with a change in perception of what the job entails.

Practitioners in a clinical speciality need regularly to see the receivers of that care, and when they separate themselves from the recipients they can become out of touch with both the women who receive care and also with the providers of care.

Doctors have a lot to learn from midwives, but one thing that they can teach us is how to stay as clinicians, even at the top of the tree. The professor of obstetrics, surgery or medicine is recognized to be an excellent clinician and as such his expertise is utilized. Once a midwife has risen above the rank of sister, she is unlikely to do any clinical practice again. Only if she has determinedly maintained her clinical involvement, often with great difficulty, against the expectations of her colleagues, the mountain of 'urgent' tasks with scant relation to the care of women, and the demands and needs of those she works with, can she maintain her clinical practice.

How could we run our service differently? Could we run it better? Someone must act as co-ordinator and there is a need for someone old and wise to act as a consultant for the less experienced practitioners. Many reading this will suggest that there is also a need to 'manage' the less able practitioner, but I would refute this suggestion. When people are given the responsibility of being autonomous and accountable, they grow into that responsibility.

Because we have adopted the nursing model which treats everyone as if they are on the lowest level of attainment, we are in danger of not allowing the most able to flower and to practise fully. Perhaps this is one reason why only one in five qualified midwives is practising, and why so many excellent midwives leave the profession to become health visitors, supervisors in Marks and Spencer, teachers or social workers.

Nursing 'procedures', showing us how to act by rote in our care of each, very individual, mother can only harm our spontaneity and ability to think creatively. Perhaps it isn't only our nurses' clothes that are harmful to midwifery. Perhaps it is many of the other aspects we have imported from the nursing field which we have taken on. How could we structure ourselves in a different way? How could we be a midwifery profession and practise as such?

Let us start at the grass roots and look at the person who is actually doing all the care now - the midwife. The midwife is a practitioner, she has learnt during her education to provide care for pregnant women, labouring women and the family during the puerperium. Each midwife works within a small team of perhaps four or six. This team has responsibility for the care of a certain number of women and the women are all booked under a particular consultant obstetrician or consultant midwife.

Because each team of midwives has responsibility for a named group of women and the care of these women depends on the midwives concerned, their sense of responsibility would be greatly increased. If a woman did not come to a clinic when she was expected, one of the midwives would make it her business to contact the woman, because she would be aware that the care of this woman depended on her and her partners.

The midwives in the team would not be community or hospital-based midwives, they would be woman-based midwives, able to go where the woman happened to be. Each team would be a team of equals, but it is likely that different members would have different skills. One would take on the responsibility of organizing the holiday rota, one would organize the time sheets and claim forms for payment, one would keep tabs on all equipment and arrange for repairs, one would take responsibility for giving thanks for the presents received.

All these professional equals would meet regularly every week to plan their work and the care of the women they are responsible for. They would report regularly to their consultant who would either be a consultant obstetrician or a consultant midwife who would also be a supervisor of midwives. The midwives attached to a consultant obstetrician would also need to relate to one of the consultant midwives who would be the supervisor of midwives for all the obstetrician-attached midwives.

The concept of a consultant midwife may seem strange, but she would be the chief clinician for women who wanted, or for whom a natural, unmedicated birth seemed appropriate. I envisage for a unit with 3000 deliveries a year that four consultant obstetricians and six consultant midwives would be required. Each consultant could have two teams of four midwives or maybe one team of six with some back-up staff in each area. The consultants would, as at present, refer to each other and all the midwives would practise their unique skills - in touch with, listening to, talking to and hand in hand with women.

Reproduced with kind permission from Nursing Time, July 10 1985

A Radical Blueprint

More home births, more community group practices, continuity of care at all times and elected supervisors of midwives. These are just some of the elements in the Association of Radical Midwives' vision of the profession's future. Caroline Flint explains

All through October packages were flying round the country and thudding on midwives' doormats. They had titles like: 'Why I am a midwife', 'What I want to be doing as a midwife in six years' time', 'How I want to see midwifery functioning in ten years' time', 'How can we manage midwifery in a creative way?' 'How much should we be paid?' 'What should a midwifery pressure group do to achieve change?' 'What are the most powerful forces/influences in midwifery today?' Every time I opened one of the envelopes, I was overwhelmed by the caring and the commitment to mothers and the midwifery profession that the documents represented. They also represented the painstaking preparation for a weekend organized by the Association of Radical Midwives to plan the future of our profession: where we wanted to go and what we wanted to achieve.

What came out of that weekend was a document called *Draft proposal for the future of the maternity services*, which is now out for consultation.

The document is mind-blowing. It begins: 'We have set out in ARM to propose a new vision for the maternity services in ten years' time. Though we recognize and applaud the strides our profession has made over the previous ten years, we feel the crisis is far from over. Many midwives feel frustrated with the present segmented pattern of maternity care and find themselves far from feeling like "practitioners in their own right".'

The new proposals are based on the following basic principles:
• The parturient woman is the central person in the process of care.

• All women should have continuity of care, whether they are at low or high risk.
• Care should be community-based.
• Women should have choice in childbirth
• Services should be accountable to the consumer.

The Association of Radical Midwives sees midwives of the future working in community group practices of between two and five midwives, and taking responsibility for the 80 per cent of women at low obstetric risk. These group practices would work from a variety of places including shops, consulting rooms, health centres, houses, community centres or local hospitals. Each group practice would take on no more than 50 women per midwife per year. These women would be cared for in the community during the antenatal period, and at home or occasionally in hospital during labour and postnatally. The midwives would be paid by the NHS, but they would be self-employed like general practitioners.

Forty per cent of midwives would work in hospital in teams of about seven attached to a consultant, caring for women at high obstetric risk. Together they would do all antenatal, intra partum and postnatal care, mainly within the hospital, but would be able to go out into the community whenever needed. They would be looking after 20 per cent of expectant mothers.

The midwives would elect their supervisor of midwives, who would be their spokesperson. She would initiate regular, frequent meetings with a representative from each group practice and each consultant-based team. She would provide information and opportunities for further education, study days, refresher courses and regular annual weekend study events. She would investigate any complaints and would organise any disciplinary hearings.

Hospital consultant obstetricians would work closely with their trusted team of midwives. They would remain, as now, the expert on the abnormal. Together with their registrar, they would have regular meetings with their midwives. The senior house officer would be seen and would see himself as a learner, and he, together with medical students and midwifery students, would be taught about midwifery matters by midwives. The student midwife would do a three-year direct entrant training course. For two years she would receive a grant as a student, and for the third year she would receive a salary.

All women would expect and receive continuity of care - there would be no place for one health professional to provide just one part of the continuum. So a GP could not pro-vide only antenatal care, but he could decide to look after women all the way through and provide all antenatal, delivery and postnatal care in the same way as the group practice midwives do. Alternatively, he might want to branch out into pre-pregnancy care, counselling and follow-up family planning.

The Radical Midwives' document also addresses itself to the issues of a midwives' trade union, the statutory bodies, practice managers, sabbaticals, international links, independent midwives, evaluation tools and so on. Here are the thoughts, dreams and aspirations of a group of committed midwives. They are determined to make it happen. If they do, midwifery will never be the same, and having a baby will be a much more pleasant experience for the majority of women in this country.

Reproduced with kind permission from Nursing Times, January 1 1986

A Different Face Each Time

What have our children's education, going to the dentist and booking a dozen driving lessons got to do with midwifery practice? Caroline Flint reveals all, in a salutary lesson on continuity of care

Education is our most precious gift to our children - yet it is the aspect of parenting that has caused me more anguish and agony than any other. Like most caring parents we looked around at all the different schools available to our children - we chose the ones we thought would best fit the needs of the particular child. We encouraged each piece of work, we exclaimed over each piece of homework, we encouraged and assisted (when we were able to understand). We went to every parents' evening and tried to support every school activity, every sale, every outing, every fund-raising event. In fact we behaved like all the other parents who are reading this piece, as most caring parents behave when faced with the enormous responsibility of educating the adults of the future.

We hung on to every word the teacher said about our little darling. If she said 'He's a nice boy', we were in ecstasies. If it was: 'She's very uncooperative', we felt like all-time failures. And then there's the influences they have - 'Miss says you shouldn't send me to school with a cold; Sir says that Spurs will win the cup; Miss says could you please make sure I have a new gym skirt for after half term'. Oh, the agony of it all. I'm so glad that they are now too old for school.

Let us look at an another aspect of education. Just imagine that when your child comes home from school, she says: 'We had a teacher called Miss Roberts today, she taught us about the fire of London'. Puzzled, I'd say: 'But you did the fire of London last week.' The child replies: 'Yes, but that was Mr Jones, Miss Roberts didn't know we had done it already. We've done France three times this term with different teachers'. Just imagine your child having a different teacher each day - having a series of supply teachers, never the same one twice. How would you feel? Would you complain? Would you try to improve the situation?

That's an extreme example. Imagine instead, going to the dentist with toothache and having a series of treatments. You were treated by Miss Jones, a very pleasant Australian woman who discussed what she was going to do. For your second treatment you find that you are to be treated by Mr Smith, an elderly and rather abrupt man, who hardly speaks to you. For your final treatment it may well be Mr Singh who tells you that instead of this being your last treatment, you have to come back again.

Imagine booking 12 driving lessons and ending up with a different instructor each week - each emphasizing different aspects of driving. If you complain to the manager of the driving school he says you are being difficult and that everyone else manages with a different instructor each time. You ring another driving school and ask them about their instructors - yes, they have 12 and you are likely to have each one if you have 12 lessons, but don't worry they all work to the same policy, they all try to say the same things.

I hope these examples are ringing bells. I am, of course, trying to give an example of what it is like for most women having a baby in 1986 in most maternity units. Research into the Know Your Midwife scheme on providing continuous care by one midwife showed that many women in the control group coming for 14 visits to the antenatal clinic saw 12 different care-givers and some saw 14. They never saw the same person twice. When they went into labour, they met more care-givers, and all this at a time of heightened awareness, heightened sensitivity, when they were feeling vulnerable and fearful. Is it right? Is it inhumane? Or just inexcusable?

I was sitting in an antenatal class one Monday evening and one of the prospective fathers said something. When I had answered, he said very perceptively: 'Of course, we wouldn't need to ask you half these questions if we knew which midwife was going to be with us during labour.'

How right he was. If he and his partner knew which midwife was going to be with them during labour they could discuss directly with the midwife how she felt about the aspects of labour they are most concerned about; what she feels about episiotomies, sytometrine and epidurals; if she will deliver the baby onto it's mother's tummy and leave the cord until it has stopped pulsating, if she is happy to leave the membranes unruptured unless there is some strong reason for rupturing them.

How hard it is for parents when you never see the same person twice, when you hear a midwife saying: 'I don't like to think of these intense relationships with parents. I like to think I work in a team, which includes obstetricians, physiotherapists, health visitors, nursery nurses, auxiliaries, domestics and students. We all say the same, we all work to the same policy."

Remember the 12 different driving instructors, and imagine what this team would be like for the woman on the receiving end. In the Know Your Midwife research we found that 43 per cent of women in the control group had 3-4 different midwives with them in labour and these were different from those they had met antenatally.

One observation made in a study of pregnant women was: 'She would like, if possible, to have someone around during labour who had given her some antenatal care.'[1] Isn't it time we recognized the inadequacies of our fragmented system and made sure that women have continuity of personnel during the childbirth continuum?

Reference

Micklethwaite, L., Beard, R., Shaw, K. (1978). 'Expectations of a pregnant woman in relation to her treatment.' *British Medical Journal* ; 2: p.188.

Reproduced with kind permission from Nursing Times, May 14, 1986

The 'Know Your Midwife' Scheme

The logistics of this enterprising scheme, which was designed to improve communication and care in pregnancy, are reviewed

The 'Know Your Midwife' scheme was conducted at St George's Hospital, Tooting from April 1983 until August 1985 - it was a scheme designed to combat the very real complaint of pregnant women going through the usual GP/community midwife/hospital doctors/hospital doctors/hospital midwives 'I never see the same face twice' syndrome. Four midwives (who happened to be hospital based) undertook the responsibility for caring for 250 women a year, they agreed to provide all antenatal care - referring women to a hospital doctor if any complication developed and having an agreement to refer all women to their consultant obstetrician at 36 weeks of pregnancy. One of the four would be with the woman throughout her labour and the four would provide the provide the bulk of postnatal care. The whole idea was that the women cared for in this way would get to know 'their' four midwives and would have the security of knowing that at whatever stage of the childbirth continuum they were, they would have a care giver they knew with them.

The 'Know Your Midwives' started by inviting women to join their scheme by letter. With the letter they sent a photo of the four of them - with details about themselves underneath the photo - whether they were married, had children, liked sport, enjoyed music, where they lived, their interests - all this was designed as a way to help the women in their care get to know the midwives better, and it also seemed to put the relationship on a more even keel. If I know intimate details about you, such as whether you have ever had a termination that no-one else knows about, or whether you regularly get cystitis - it seems only fair that you should know something more about me, even if it is very non-threatening information such as the names of my children and that I like going to the theatre. The four midwives worked a rota which mainly had two duties - the early shift when the midwife would be on duty from 8am, when the midwife would come to the postnatal ward and do postnatal nursings on the women from the scheme (usually about four women) and then she would go out into the community and do postnatal checks on women from the scheme who had gone home (she would see approximately four women), meanwhile the women on the ward would be looked after by the regular postnatal ward staff. The midwife on early shift would then come back to the hospital to run an antenatal clinic at which she would see five to six women at half hourly intervals. If she ever needed to refer a woman to a doctor, the clinic was in the hospital and she could just bleep whoever was on call. The midwife on an early shift came off duty whenever she had finished which was normally between 4 and 5 pm, but at weekends was more likely to be about 1.30 - 2 pm because no antenatal clinic was held at the weekends.

The other duty the 'Know Your Midwives' worked was an 'On Call' shift which lasted from 7.45 am until 7.45 am the following day - a full 24 hours. The midwife on call would carry a bleep and she would be on call from her home - the 'Know Your

Midwives' were on call seven times every three weeks and they reckoned that for three of those periods they would not be called at all, but of course this was not guaranteed and some midwives seemed to be always called and others hardly ever. If the 'Know Your Midwife' was not called by a woman in labour/with a query/wanting to change her advance) and get to know each other very well, this enabled a very supportive and cherishing atmosphere to develop. Each midwife kept a record of the amount of time she had worked, if she was on call but not called, she would write down three hours for that day if she went to the postnatal ward from 4 - 7 pm. If the midwife was called to antenatal appointment/worried about the baby, she would only come into the hospital from 4 - 7 pm when she would check and help the postnatal women from the scheme in the postnatal ward, she would also do any community evening visits that needed doing.

MONTH BEGINNING: ______ HOSPITAL: ______

S	M	Tu	W	Th	F	S	S	M	Tu	W	Th	F	S	S	M	Tu	W	Th	F	S	S	M	Tu	W	Th	F	S
AL	AL	AL	AL	AL	AL	AL	D	D	D	OC	E	OC	½	OC	E	OC	E	D	D	OC	½	D	D	OC	E	X	OC
OC	E	OC	E	D	D	OC	½	OC	E	1-9	OC	E	D	D	D	D	OC	E	OC	½	OC	E	OC	E	D	D	X
½	OC	E	1-9	OC	E	D	AL	AL	AL	AL	AL	AL	AL	AL	AL	AL	AL	AL	AL	AL	X	OC	E	1-9	OC	E	D
D	D	D	OC	E	OC	½	OC	E	OC	E	D	D	OC	½	OC	E	1-9	OC	E	D	D	D	D	X	X	OC	½

Fig. I

On a Wednesday was a duty which was worked on that day and no other - 1-9 pm, when the midwife would come in to do an antenatal clinic which ran from 1.15 - 9 pm and at which she would see 19 women with 20 minute appointments, with the 'Know Your Midwife' working on an early shift who saw five to six women, between them they saw 25 antenatal women. The clinic on Wednesdays had a break in it from 4.30 - 6 pm when all the 'Know Your Midwives' would gather, have a cup of tea, eat mountains of chocolates and discuss women they were concerned about, women they were due to deliver and what sort of labour and care they were hoping for, they also took this opportunity to exchange ideas, swap off duty (which they knew for about six months in someone at 8 am and worked through until 8 pm with only a half-hour break, she would write down 11.5 hours, at the end of the month all the hours were totalled and those midwives who had worked more than 150 hours in a 28 day period were repaid their time. In the sample of duty (Figure 1) the spaces marked X are when midwives are being paid time back. OC = On Call. E = Early Shift, a half = early shift which finishes early, D = Day Off, AL = Annual Leave.

Alongside the operation of 'Know Your Midwife' scheme a research project was set up to evaluate what happened to women looked after almost exclusively by midwives who they had been able to get to know. Women were looked after in labour by someone they knew and this was much appreciated.

Reproduced with kind permission from Midwife, Health Visitor and Community Nurse, May 1986

In Search of Continuity of Care

In midwifery the newest 'buzz' word is 'the team approach' – wherever you happen to go the midwives are trying to achieve, or indeed have achieved, a 'team approach' to care. And this phrase is thought to incorporate all that is good in maternity care: the team approach is better for women, the team approach is better for midwives. Or is it? Could it just be a meaningless phrase?

The team approach was coined as a synonym for 'continuity of care.' Many of us see that working a thirty seven and a half week it is impossible for a midwife to provide continuity of care on her own. Women need to form a relationship with a small group of midwives in order to achieve the desired effect of having someone you know, throughout the whole continuum of pregnancy, labour, delivery and the postnatal period.

Some schemes along those lines have been set up – the aim being that women and midwives could form a meaningful relationship throughout the whole continuum. The team of midwives has taken responsibility for the care of a specified number of women: they are 'women based', their care is organized around the women and they are peripatetic.

Other teams have been set up based on a ward model. A consultant obstetrician usually heads the team and the midwives work on a ward. They identify themselves as a cohesive group and call themselves a team, they feel more united and enjoy being together more because they feel that they have a common purpose and a common aim.

Minority

When women are admitted to the ward antenatally they get to know the midwives who care for them before and after the delivery. The theory is that the midwives from the ward go to the delivery suite and deliver the women they know. The woman who has been an inpatient antenatally sometimes has this sort of care and for her it is very pleasant – but women who are admitted antenatally are a tiny minority. What happens to the women who remain healthy throughout their pregnancy? What happens to the vast majority of women?

The theory is that these women will meet one of the midwives from their team at some time when they are visiting the antenatal clinic. The ward tries to send a midwife from the ward to the antenatal clinic each time 'their' consultant has a clinic. But logistically the chances of the woman meeting and being able to have a meaningful discussion with that midwife is small if the same midwife has to help in a clinic seeing anything up to 100 women.

If the woman goes to the clinic in the hospital a total of five times throughout her pregnancy she has a chance of catching a glimpse of one of the midwives from her team on five occasions. She may even have a meaningful conversation with one of those midwives or even two.

Labour

When the woman goes into labour the chances of her being looked after throughout her labour by one of those two midwives – or even one of those five midwives – are very slim. She is much more likely to be looked after by a midwife she has never met before. Even if the midwife feels at one with the woman, even if her best friend is the team midwife that the woman met in the antenatal clinic, for the woman she is a stranger.

Some postnatal wards run on 'team lines'. You can go into postnatal wards across the country and see midwives from team A and team B – only to discover that they work in two separate teams.

Hopefully they care for the same woman today as they cared for yesterday. But if the midwife had a day off yesterday and the woman is going home tomorrow morning 'continuity of care' in this situation can mean meeting the woman for a couple of short snatches. As far as the woman is concerned she is still being surrounded by strange faces at this vulnerable time in her life.

I have looked hard at these attempts at continuity of care and it seems to me that the flaw in them is that they are based around the institution and the basic set up of that institution. No attempt is made to change the institution and the midwives are scurrying around trying to achieve something else while actually not changing anything as far as the woman is concerned.

It seems to me that we have to change the emphasis. Once the woman is seen as the paramount individual, once the care is centred on her and her needs (expressed time and time again over the last decade as 'wanting to have someone with her in labour who she had been able to get to know during the antenatal period') the emphasis changes. No longer is the institution seen as paramount.

Woman centred

It is the woman who is paramount. We can then arrange care to be woman-centred and a small team of midwives takes responsibility for a small group of women.

When the woman goes into labour those midwives take responsibility for being there and will usually have developed a type of 'on call' system. After the baby is born the midwives will care for the woman as each day passes.

She knows them all, she has made a relationship with them – they are not just midwives she has caught a glimpse of across a crowded antenatal clinic or smiled at across a 'tea party', She has really *got to know* her midwives.

At the moment 'the team approach' is meaningless as far as women are concerned. We might just as well say we are using the 'Monte Carlo method' or the 'Viggins Routine' – meaningless phrases, we have to do better than this.

Reproduced with kind permission from Primary Health Care, October 1987.

How the Midwife's Role Needs to Change

Caroline Flint is an independent midwife, currently looking for a post in the Health Service where she can set up teams of midwives so that all women will know the midwives who are with her throughout pregnancy, labour and the postnatal period. She is associate midwifery editor of Nursing Times

Most women (76 per cent) in this country are delivered by midwives. Women have been asking for a long time to be able to get to know those attendants who will be with them during labour - they do not want to have strangers with them when they are giving birth. This desire for continuity affects many aspects of our lives - we tend to buy our groceries at the same store, we tend to go to the same bank, the same garage to have our car repaired, the same hairdresser. We find security and comfort in having the same people dealing with our needs and often it is more efficient: if I always see the same doctor I do not have to explain what happened when this illness started: if I go to the same dentist every time he knows whether I like an injection of local anaesthetic before he even asks me to open my mouth or that I do not want an injection whatever happens. Childbirth is not only one of life's most intimate experiences but also a hugely life-changing experience, so continuity is even more important than in routine and everyday happenings in our lives.

Women have been telling us this for at least the past decade and saying how important continuity of carer is for them in childbirth.

1978
Micklethwaite, Beard and Shaw
'She would like, if it were possible, to have someone around during her labour who had given her some antenatal care.'

1980
Short Report
'I think this is what women complain about most: they do not have continuity of care which they want very much during their antenatal visits but certainly during labour and delivery.'

'We recognize the difficulties of providing continuity of care throughout pregnancy and labour but consider that a measure of it can be obtained by better organization.'

1981
Kitzinger
'There is an almost complete absence of continuity of care and each time she attends a woman sees different, anonymous faces.'

1982
MSAC
'Continuity of care. It is important that the woman should be able to build up a relationship of trust with the staff she meets, and efforts should be made to involve the same group of staff at each visit.'

1982
Boyd and Sellers
'I was more relaxed because my midwife was with me.'

'By and large it is the midwife who makes or breaks a happy delivery.'

'These women enjoyed labour - they were given choice, they were attended by midwives they liked.'

'My labour was a truly delightful experience attended by professional people that I regarded as friends.'

1982
Royal College of Obstetricians and Gynaecologists
'It has been suggested to us that women should have the same midwife to attend them in labour as in the antenatal period. We consider this continuity of care to be an ideal aim and it may be possible in some circumstances.'

1983
Ong, Family Service Units
'Plan effective continuity of care - women should have the opportunity of building up a relationship with one doctor, one midwife.'

1983
PARENTS survey to which 7,500 women replied
'Mothers would like antenatal, delivery and postnatal care to be provided, as far as possible, by the same people. Again and again, letters expressed the anxiety that arises when seeing a different doctor at each visit to the antenatal clinic, and at being delivered by total strangers - sometimes two different shifts of total strangers if a woman had a long labour.'

1986
PARENTS survey to which 9,000 women replied
'Good communications between parents and the medical staff were helped where women saw the same doctor and midwife regularly - most mothers saw different people at almost every antenatal visit and were delivered by total strangers. While full of praise for the care they received, many women wished they could have had more continuity of care through pregnancy and beyond.'

In a survey looking at 577 women receiving shared care with their general practitioners from Spring 1983 until Spring 1985, Flint and Poulengeris found that women having shared care found their GPs friendly and appearing to take a personal interest in the woman and her pregnancy. 85.4 per cent of women having shared care were satisfied with their antenatal care and would have chosen that type of antenatal care again. When they looked back on their labours six weeks later they did not perceive it as such a wonderful or enjoyable experience as a group of women who had received care from a continuous group of midwives all the way through pregnancy, labour and the postnatal period. They did not feel as much in control of the situation, nor did they feel so prepared for motherhood or find being a mother so easy as the groups who had full hospital care.

The authors of the report conclude that those women who opt for what is now the most common type of arrangement - shared care with a GP - do not have such a happy birth experience and miss out afterwards also. They suggest that a GP should feel more able to go and see his patient in the labour ward, and also that a GP should work with a small team of midwives during pregnancy, one of whom would be with the woman during labour. This would mean that she would have someone from 'outside' with her in the hospital whilst she is in labour. This last suggestion is echoed in the Association of Radical Midwives Discussion Document 'The Vision' and the Royal College of Midwives Document 'The Role and Education of the Future Midwife in the United Kingdom' who both recommend that midwives should work in small teams and take responsibility for providing continuity of care for a specific group of women: women have been asking us for this for long enough - it is time we started to respond to their pleas.

References

Association of Radical Midwives.(1986). *'The Vision - Proposals for the future of the maternity services.'*

Boyd, C., Sellars, L., (1982). *'The British Way of Birth.'* Pan Books Ltd.

Flint, C., Poulengeris, P. (1987).'The Know Your Midwife Report.'

HMSO (1979-80) 'Second Report from the Social Services Committee. Session , Perinatal and Neonatal Mortality.' June, HMSO.

Kitzinger, S. (1981). 'Change in Antenatal Care.' A report of a working party set up for the National Childbirth Trust. National Childbirth Trust.

Maternity Services Advisory Committee (1982). 'Maternity care in action. Part 1 - Antenatal Care.' Crown Copyright.

Micklethwaite, P., Beard, R., Shaw, K. (1978). 'Expectations of a Pregnant woman in relation to her treatment.' *British Medical Journal.* 1978;2: pp.188-91.

Oakley, A. (1980). 'Women Confined.' Oxford: Martin Robertson, .

Ong, Bie Nio. (1983). 'Our Motherhood.' Family Service Units, 207 Old Marylebone Road, London NW1 5QP.

Parents Magazine.(1983). 'Birth in Britain. A Parents special report.' p.92.

Parents Magazine. 'BIRTH 9000 mothers speak out. Birth Survey 19896 - results.' 1986; p.128.

Royal College of Midwives (1987). 'The Role and Education of the Future Midwife in the United Kingdom'.

Royal College of Obstetricians and Gynaecologists (1982). 'Report of the RCOG working party on antenatal and intrapartum care.'

Reproduced with kind permission from Maternal and Child Health, December, 1987

Know Your Midwife

Five years ago, a team of midwives from South London set out to develop a new breed of midwife - one who would tend to mothers both at home and in hospital. This week, Caroline Flint reports on the findings of the scheme, which could have a major impact on the future of midwifery

Between April 1983 and August 1985 at St George's Hospital, South London, a group of midwives calling themselves the Know Your Midwife Team took responsibility for 250 pregnant women each year for two years. To evaluate the effect of their ministrations a randomized controlled trial was set up with the criteria for women entered in the trial being:

• Over 5ft tall
• No serious medical conditions
• No previous uterine surgery
• No more than two miscarriages or terminations of pregnancy
• No previous intrauterine growth retardation
• No previous stillborn babies or neonatal deaths
• No previous preterm labours
• No Rhesus antibodies

The trial was conducted because so much that is done in maternity care has been completely unevaluated. A randomized controlled trial is a fair and easy way of evaluating the effect of treatment on a certain population compared with a control group which does not receive the intervention.

The women in the control group received normal hospital care and because both groups were chosen randomly it was possible to compare the women's responses and see the effect of care from a group of midwives whom the women had got to know.

The total number of women studied for this trial was 1,001; 503 were in the Know Your Midwife group (KYM) and 498 women were in the control group. The controls received normal hospital care during their pregnancy, labour and puerperium. The KYM group received antenatal care from four midwives. The midwives saw the women at every antenatal visit except for the first booking visit, and at 36 weeks and 41 weeks of pregnancy when they saw either a consultant obstetrician or a senior registrar.

The trial was designed to show whether a KYM system was feasible; whether the KYM women actually saw less care givers than the control group, what the women thought about the care they received, whether it was cost-effective and whether the obstetric outcome of the two groups showed any differences.

The results of the trial showed that women seeing midwives on the Know Your Midwife Scheme really did see less care givers during their pregnancy and labour and in labour they were invariably looked after by a midwife they had got to know during pregnancy.

Women's satisfaction with the care they received was evaluated by three questionnaires given to them at 37 weeks antenatally and two days then six weeks postnatally. In terms of emotional satisfaction the women who were offered Know Your Midwife care fared much more positively than the control group. In the antenatal clinic only 15 per cent of the KYM group reported a usual waiting time of more than half an hour compared with 71 per cent in the control group. In the antenatal clinic, the KYM group overall seemed happier with their care. They felt that they were encouraged to ask questions more than women in the control group. They felt that the midwives appeared interested in them as a person and that they helped with anxieties more than the women in the control group.

It could be suggested that because the KYM group midwives were able to build a relationship with the women they were seeing, the women in turn found it easier to voice their anxieties and felt more able to talk to the midwives. Over the past decade psychologists have highlighted the importance of establishing a good rapport with patients. This encourages the disclosure of important problems which are often more social than medical. Midwives would certainly be able to enhance rapport if they had the advantage of repeated consultations with the same women.

Regarding women's expectations for labour, more of the women in the KYM group wanted to be 'active' during labour than women in the control group and in fact this is what happened. The KYM group walked about more in labour than women in the control group. More than half of the KYM group reported being able to choose their position during labour. Significantly more of the KYM group gave birth in alternative positions compared with the control group.

At the International Congress of Psychosomatic Obstetrics and Gynaecology in 1980[1] it was suggested that being able to choose the position in labour – for example, walking, standing – increases the woman's perception of control.

The women in the Know Your Midwife group found the staff they had with them in labour more caring than the women in the control group. This is important when considering Kirke's findings[2] that there was a close association with mothers' reports of treatment and attention by staff in labour, and whether a mother would return to the same hospital for a future birth.

The babies of women in the KYM group were put to the breast sooner than babies of the control group mothers. As would be expected from the work of Salaryia[3], more babies of the KYM group mothers were breastfeeding at six weeks. This was not statistically significant.

Women's feelings about their labours six weeks later differed significantly between the two groups. More of the KYM group women remembered their labours as wonderful or enjoyable and fewer of them looked back on their labours as dreadful or not enjoyable.

The KYM women felt that all choices in labour were always explained to them, and that the midwives with them always explained what the were doing. Good communications between staff and mothers was found by Kirke to be significantly associated with overall satisfaction with care.

Postnatal ward staff were perceived as more caring by the KYM group than by the controls.

In the KYM group 72.3 per cent (180) saw postnatal staff as 'very caring' compared to 56.4 per cent (128) of the controls. Interestingly, one of the criticisms of the Know Your Midwife scheme was that the KYM midwives did not provide 24-hour care for their women in the postnatal ward. However, this seems to be outweighed by the benefits of being cared for by someone they knew.

The KYM women reported that being a mother was easier. Perhaps this was because they felt better prepared than the women in the control group.

The KYM group received continuity of midwife care with fewer carers. However the actual time with staff was not substantially greater for the KYM group than for the controls.

Huggins[4] studied a small group of the women in this project. She found that the women in both groups saw care givers for similar lengths of time. However, the control group had their care fragmented while the KYM women were seen by one midwife for an unbroken period of time.

There were some interesting differences in the obstetric outcome of the groups. Although the reasons for antenatal admissions were similar, there were pro-portionately more antenatal admissions for more than nine days in the control group. These included non-medical social admissions which sometimes were in addition to purely medical problems.

Women in the KYM group spent less time in hospital. This may reflect the person-alized care they received.

The KYM midwives also saw the women for longer in the antenatal clinic. This may have given them time to discuss prob-lems which a doctor may feel he has not time to do. The KYM midwives could also visit women at home antenatally to check blood pressure or supervise a woman at home so that she had more rest. Kowalski[5] also found that women who were offered continuity of care were admitted less frequently ante-natally.

It was expected that home visits dur-ing labour would reduce the time that wom-en spent in hospital before delivery as shown by Klein and colleagues[6]. The KYM women did have shorter stays before delivery com-pared to the controls, but the difference was not significant for primigravidae although it was significantly shorter for multigravid women. This partly confirms Klein's results.

The labour induction rate was similar in both groups, but the KYM group had sig-nificantly fewer accelerated labours than the controls. Women in the KYM group report-ed being monitored by electronic fetal mon-itoring less than the controls – 271 KYMs to 254 controls.

The difference between the groups in type of labour and monitoring may partly reflect the early management of labour. When a KYM woman went into labour she would bleep her KYM midwife on call. The midwife would be likely to know the woman's individual circumstances, especially if she had seen her at her last antenatal visit. If she did not visit her at home in labour, the KYM midwife would sometimes arrange to ring back within an hour or so for a progress report. However, when a control group woman went into labour, the labour ward staff would frequently ask her to come straight away. Thus different early labour management may partly account for the reduced use of acceleration and monitoring in the KYM group. Klein also found that women admitted later in labour had less syntocinon acceleration of labour and less electronic fetal monitoring[6].

The women in the KYM group spent 52 minutes longer in the first stage of labour (seven hours 15 minutes in the KYM group compared to six hours 23 minutes in the con-trol) although there is no difference in the length of the second stage of labour.

Chertock[7] has suggested that psycho-logical factors have a considerable role in the course of labour. The KYM women were with midwives whom they knew and may well have felt less stressed because of this. It is possible that this could have contributed to their having slightly longer labours than the controls, although the chemical pathways mediating this are uncertain. It is interesting that Shear et al[8] found that women who re-ceived more continuity of care also had longer labours than those not having any continuity (nine hours 12 minutes compared to eight hours and 24 minutes). Klein[6] found labour-ing primigravidae visited at home had sig-nificantly longer first stage labours than those who were not visited.

Despite the longer length of their first stage of labour, 51.4 per cent (246) of the KYM had no analgesia in labour compared with 38.1 per cent (180) in the control group. Women in the control group were almost twice as likely to have an epidural during labour compared with the KYM group. The KYM group had less analgesia than the controls, but were just as satisfied with their pain relief as the control group – 88.5 per cent (185) of the KYM group reported being very or fairly satisfied with pain relief compared with 83.9 per cent of the controls.

The lower epidural rate in the KYM group may have been one of the reasons that they had more normal deliveries than the control group.

The Caesarean rate was similar in both groups – 7.5 per cent (37) in the KYM group and 7.4 per cent (35) in the controls. All the women in both groups were 'low risk', therefore it is not surprising that these rates are lower than for the hospital as a whole. The overall rate of Caesareans at St George's Hospital for 1984 was 13.4 per cent (334) and for 1985 was 13.7 per cent (418).

Significantly more babies born to women in the KYM group needed no resuscitation or only mucus extraction. Fewer of the KYM group babies needed oxygen or intermittent positive pressure ventilation. On the other hand more babies in the KYM group had an Apgar score of less then seven at five minutes after birth. However, there was no significant difference between the two groups in the numbers of babies admitted to the special care baby unit.

More babies born to mothers offered KYM care were stillborn (four compared to two), or died neonatally (four compared to two), but numbers are too small to be able to examine statistical significance. Detailed case histories of all the babies show that the fact that these women were being looked after by midwives seems irrelevant. Whoever they had been looked after the outcome would almost certainly have been unchanged.

Finally, financial implications. Know Your Midwife care would seem to have been more cost effective than control care. From the women's point of view, those women who experienced KYM care waited for significantly less time in the antenatal clinic. Many of the women were working. Their absence from work would represent a financial outlay for their employer. It is obvious therefore that to have an employee away from work for a short time is more cost effective than to have that same employee away from work for a long period of time.

In a small study of costs we suggest that it was 20-25 per cent more expensive for the woman in the control group to receive their antenatal care than for the women in the KYM group. Despite having *Midwives Clinic*

stamped on the notes, women in the control group actually saw doctors more often than women in the KYM group.

This is more expensive because doctors cost more than midwives. Added to this is the fact that doctors frequently have trained personnel to assist them. They also have more support staff such as a receptionist, people to test urine and weigh the women. It is clear that the costing of the actual consultation is greater. This would be a small price to pay if the doctors were actually doing more than the midwives. But the questionnaires showed the control group women were no more reassured by doctors than by midwives.

As the control group were twice as likely to ask for epidurals this also represented savings by the KYM group. It was difficult to obtain accurate figures for costing within the NHS, so we asked the cost of an epidural plus one top-up in a local private maternity unit and we were quoted £220. However, as 55 more women in the control group had epidurals this represents a saving of £12, 100 for the KYM group at this rate. Perhaps as NHS epidural plus one top-up may not cost as much. Nevertheless the cost of providing epidural analgesia for the KYM group was still half that of the control group.

If it was beneficial for a higher number of women to have an epidural analgesia, or if the women in the KYM group had been denied the analgesia they requested this cost saving would have been at the expense of women's comfort. Quite the contrary actually is the case. Women in the KYM group appreciated the level of analgesia they received and they looked back on their labours more favourably than women in the control group.

The women having KYM care spent a total of 920 days in antenatal ward compared with the women in the control group who spent 1075 days. Although this did not reach statistical significance it did represent a cost saving of £24,800 over the two-year period.

In this study the service provided by the team of four midwives was found to give a much higher level of patient satisfaction to the group receiving it. This enabled them to face motherhood feeling much more prepared. It was feasible because the women receiving this care actually saw fewer care givers. They had someone with them during labour who had given them some antenatal care and would go on to provide postnatal care. The results obtained from this small study are consistent with women having no worse an obstetric outcome than women treated conventionally. Apparently the type of care the midwife team provided saved money, not just because midwifery personnel cost less but also because the type of care midwives provide appears to be cheaper than care currently provided for women.

This study has several implications for maternity care:

• That midwives should take over the care of low-risk women to a far greater extent than is done at the present.

• That continuity of care by a small group is feasible and preferable for women, and far greater efforts should be made to achieve it.

• That all the care givers at present involved in the care of childbearing women are useful and needed, but instead of them all seeing very little of a large number of women, the emphasis should be that each care giver sees more of fewer women. Conversely each woman should be able to know and identify with a few care givers whom she will see all the way through the childbearing continuum. This will enable the care giver to build up a relationship with the woman and the woman to build up a relationship with her care givers.

This research was carried out with a grant from the South West Thames Regional Health Authority and the Wellington Foundation. Polly Poulengeris was the research assistant. The whole project could not have been carried out without the support and involvement of all the midwives and obstetricians at St George's Hospital.

References
1. Collishaw, M.E. (1980). 'Reporting on international congress of pyschosomatic obstetrics and gynaecology in West Berlin'. *Midwives Chronicle*. March 1981, p.91.
2. Kirke, P.N. (1980). 'Mothers view of care in labour'. *British Journal of Obstetrics and Gynaecology*, 87, pp.1034-1037.
3. Salariya, E.M., Easton, P.M., Carter, J.I. (1987). 'Duration of breastfeeding after early initiation wand frequent feeding.' *The Lancet,* November 25th, pp.1141-1143.
4. Huggins, C. (1985). 'A comparative study of two antenatal care systems in terms of waiting time and encounters.' Unpublished BSc. dissertation Dept. of Nursing, Chelsea College, London.
5. Kowalski, K., Gottschalk, J., Greer, B., Watson, A., Bowes, J.R. (1977). 'Team nursing coverage of prenatal – intrapartum patients in a university hospital.' *British Journal of Obstetrics and Gynaecology* 50 (1), pp.116-119.
6. Klein, M., Lloyd, I., Redman, C., Bull, M., Turnbull, A.C. (1983). 'A comparison of low-risk women booked for delivery in two different systems of care.' *British Journal of Obstetrics and Gynaecology*. 90, pp.118–128.
7. Chertok, L. (1971). 'Psychosomatic aspects of childbirth.' In Morris, N. (Ed). *Psychosomatic Medicine in Obstetrics and Gynaecology.* 3rd International Congress: London.
8. Shear, C.L., Gipe, B.T., Mattheis, J.K., Levy, N. (1983). 'Provider continuity and quality of medical care.' *Medical Care* 21(12), pp.1204-1210.

Reproduced with kind permission from Nursing Times, September 21 1988.

The Know Your Midwife Scheme

A randomized trial of continuity of care by a team of midwives

A team of four midwives provided the care during pregnancy, labour and the puerperium to 503 women at low obstetric risk, over a two-year period. Compared with standard hospital care randomly allocated to 498 women this 'Know Your Midwife' scheme was associated with greater continuity in all phases of maternity care. The scheme appeared very acceptable to women: they spent less time in the antenatal clinic, and overall, felt more satisfied, better prepared and better able to discuss problems. The scheme was characterized by less obstetric intervention particularly in respect of augmentation of labour and intrapartum analgesia; labours tended to be longer. Neonatal outcome was generally similar in the two groups but the size of the trial did not allow a precise assessment of differential effects in these terms. The 'Know Your Midwife' scheme is feasible. It should now be introduced more widely but in a way which allows continuing evaluation.

Introduction

The care received by many women during pregnancy, labour and puerperium is fragmented and lacking in continuity (Royal College of Obstetricians and Gynaecologists, 1982). The distress which this can cause is well recognized and there have been calls for changes in the organization of perinatal care (Social Services Committee, 1980; Association of Radical Midwives, 1986; Royal College of Midwives, 1987) so that a woman 'can build up a relationship of trust with the staff she meets' (Maternity Services Advisory Committee, 1982). The Maternity Services Advisory Committee , for example, has suggested that 'efforts should be made to involve the same group of staff at each visit' and 'ideally', 'women should have the same midwife to attend them in labour as in antenatal period' (Maternity Services Advisory Committee, 1982).

The 'Know Your Midwife' scheme was established at St George's Hospital, London, in 1983 to try and meet these ideals. The in-tention was that a team of four midwives would give continuity of care during pregnancy, labour and the puerperium to 250 women each year, with the back up of the hospital obstetricians. Suitability for inclusion in this scheme, of women who wished to have all their care at the hospital, would be assessed after review of the past medical history and first physical examination. Thereafter most care would be given by the team of four midwives but an obstetrician would be consulted routinely at 36 and 41 weeks of pregnancy (if applicable) and at any other time when the midwife requested it.

To evaluate the scheme it was introduced in the context of a randomized controlled trial. The findings of this study are summarized here. A more detailed report (Flint and Poulengeris, 1986) is available on request from one of us (CF).

There were two main purposes of this study. The first was to assess whether the provision of total perinatal care by a team of four midwives is feasible and does, indeed, result in greater continuity of care. The latter was measured by the number of caregivers seen during pregnancy and labour and whether women had met their intrapartum caregiver during pregnancy. The second was to assess the scheme's acceptability to women at low obstetric risk. The differential effects of the two policies on the clinical management and outcome of perinatal care were also examined, but it was recognized in advance that a trial of the size envisaged would provide only imprecise estimates of these, particularly in respect of relatively uncommon adverse outcomes.

Methods

The trial was conducted at St George's Hospital, London. Women 'booking' for delivery at the hospital between April 1983 and March 1985 were considered for entry if they were likely to receive their full antenatal care at the hospital. The reasons for attending the hospital for all care were either the general practitioner did not offer 'shared care' or the women preferred to attend the hospital. The entry criteria were:
• the woman was over five feet tall (132 cm)
• she had no serious medical problems
• there had been no previous uterine surgery
• there was no past obstetric history of more than two miscarriages or terminations of pregnancy, or of stillbirth or neonatal death, or of a baby with intrauterine growth retardation or preterm delivery
• there were no Rhesus antibodies in the cur rent pregnancy.

After the first visit to the hospital, women who met these criteria of low risk were then randomly allocated, using sealed opaque envelopes, to one of two forms of hospital- based care. Four hundred and ninety eight women received the hospital's standard antenatal, intrapartum and postpartum care for low risk women. The other group (503 women) were sent a letter offering antenatal, intrapartum and postpartum care by a team of four midwives as part of the 'Know Your Midwife' scheme (Flint, 1986). Forty

three (nine per cent) declined; in practice these women received the standard form of hospital care but for the purpose of analysis they have been retained in the 'Know Your Midwife' group to avoid selection bias. The final sample size was dictated by the maximum length of time (two years) that recruitment could continue.

All data were collected in the same ways for both groups. Clinical data on all the women in the trial were transcribed from the casenotes after delivery. The casenotes of all 101 women booked to deliver in a 2-month period during the trial were studied in greater detail to describe the caregivers who were actually seen by the women.

Assessment of maternal satisfaction was limited to the final 559 women recruited in the trial. A standardized questionnaire was given out at 37 weeks of pregnancy to 285 women in the 'Know Your Midwife' group and to 274 women in the control group; this was returned by 277 (97 per cent) and 268 (98 per cent) respectively. Further questionnaires were distributed at two days and six weeks after delivery to 279 women and 267 women (for compassionate reasons women whose baby was in the Special Care Nursery were not included). The first of these perinatal questionnaires was returned by 275 (99 per cent) and 261 (98 per cent) women, and the second by 249 (89 per cent) and 227 (85 per cent) women. Where appropriate, the source of data is indicated on the Tables. Clinical outcome data are not available for 15 women allocated to the 'Know Your Midwife' scheme and for 19 women in the control group because they moved away during pregnancy. Individual items are missing for a few women in both the casenotes and questionnaire datasets and this is why the denominators vary slightly.

Chi square and Student's 't' statistical tests were used as appropriate. Confidence intervals of the relative rates were calculated using the method recommended by Morris and Gardner (1988), 99 per cent rather than 95 per cent intervals are presented because of the many comparisons made between the groups. The confidence interval gives a range in which the true effect is likely to lie. If the 99 per cent confidence interval does not include unity the difference between the two groups is statistically significant at the one per cent level (p<0.01).

Findings

The two groups derived by random allocation were similar at entry in most respects (Table 1); there were, however , more Asian women in the control group and more smokers in the 'Know Your Midwife' group.

The 'Know Your Midwife' scheme was associated with greater continuity of care (Table 2). Fewer caregivers were seen during pregnancy. During labour, the 'Know Your Midwife' group saw both fewer midwives and fewer doctors (Table 2). The caregiver during labour already known to the women in the standard care group was usually a junior doctor whom they had met in the antenatal clinic; the caregiver known to the women in the 'Know Your Midwife' group was invariably one of the four 'Know Your Midwife' midwives who stayed with the women throughout labour.

The 'Know Your Midwife' scheme appeared to be more acceptable to the women in almost every aspect investigated. Some of the parameters which differed between the groups are described in Table 3. In the antenatal clinic there were fewer delays, easier discussion of anxieties and greater satisfaction generally. Two days after the delivery, women in the 'Know Your Midwife' group were more likely to feel that they had been well prepared for labour and to rate those who had been looked after them during labour as 'very caring'. Six weeks after delivery there were striking differences in the women's recollection of labour, about their preparedness for child care and the ease with which they could discuss problems during their puerperium.

Clinically, the 'Know Your Midwife' scheme was charecterized by less obstetric intervention (Table 4). The difference in the rates of augmentation, epidural and intramuscular analgesia and episiotomy were statistically significant. Overall, rates of perineal trauma were, however, almost identical because of a reciprocal increase in vaginal tears in the 'Know Your Midwife' group. The tendency for labours to be longer in the ' Know Your Midwife' group may be related to the difference in augmentation of labour, but could also be due to a different definition of the onset of labour.

Neonatal outcome was generally similar in the two groups (Table 5). There were more low five minute Apgar scores in the 'Know Your Midwife' group but neonatal resuscitation was used significantly less often in this group and the final status on the delivery suite was similar as judged by the numbers of babies who were transferred to the Special Care Nursery. There were four stillbirths and four neonatal deaths in the 'Know Your Midwife' group compared with two stillbirths and two neonatal deaths in the standard care group. Review of these 12 cases by an experienced obstetrician suggests that it is unlikely that any could have been prevented by a change in care. With such a small number of events the confidence intervals are wide (Table 5) and include both a clinically important increase and a clinically important decrease in the risk of perinatal death associated with the 'Know Your Midwife' scheme.

Secondary analyses showed that adjustment for ethnicity and smoking makes no statistically significant difference to these findings. Women of European origin were more likely to have an epidural and less likely to have pethidine analgesia. These adjustments tended to accentuate the contrast between the groups in epidural use and slightly reduce the difference in pethidine use.

Discussion

The experiment has shown that a team of four midwives successfully cared for 500 women at low obstetric risk over a two-year period.

Table 1. Socio-demographic characteristics of the trial groups

	Know Your Midwife	Standard
	n = 503	n = 498
Mean [SD] maternal age	25.8 [5.1]	25.4 [5.0]
No. (%) primiparous	288 (57)	291 (58)
No. (%) married	368 (76)	371 (78)
Ethnic group: No. (%)		
Caucasian	367 (73)	311 (63)
Asian	48 (10)	90 (18)
Afro-caribbean	74 (15)	74 (15)
Other	14 (3)	20 (4)
	n = 277*	n = 268*
No. (%) smokers	83 (30)	59 (22)
No. (%) in paid employment at 37 weeks' gestation	20 (7)	18 (7)
Housing: No. (%)		
Own home	142 (51)	136 (51)
Rented	88 (32)	87 (32)
Other	47 (17)	45 (17)

* Respondents to 37-week questionnaire

The trial provided clear evidence that the 'Know Your Midwife' scheme as practised at St George's hospital during 1983 to 1985 did improve continuity of care and was more acceptable to women at low obstetric risk than the standard hospital care. The 'Know Your Midwife' policy was also associated with a reduction in obstetric intervention, particularly in respect of augmentation of labour and intrapartum analgesia. The lower rates of episiotomy and instrumental delivery are also similar to the findings of the only two comparable controlled trials (Runnerstrom, 1969; Slome et al, 1976) identified from the Oxford Database of Perinatal Trials (Chalmers et al, 1986). There were however, more tears in the experimental group of the trial and the overall trauma rates were identical.

The difference in the five-minute Apgar scores is likely to reflect the difference in the use of neonatal resuscitation; the rates of admission to the Special Care Nursery do not suggest a major adverse effect of the 'Know Your Midwife' policy on pregnancy outcome. Although there were more deaths in the 'Know Your Midwife' group the total number is small and the confidence interval is very wide; as recognized at the outset, the trial was too small to assess with any precision the safety of the scheme in terms of perinatal mortality.

The scheme does demand extra responsibility from the midwives and this change in practice was sometimes stressful, particularly at first, for both those implementing the scheme and those administering it. The provision of continuity of care over a 24-hour-period also meant that occasionally a midwife worked for long hours without formal back-up at nights or at the weekends. Expansion of the team to five or six midwives would allow a second midwife 'on call' and greater flexibility in the rota, although this would probably reduce continuity. The four midwives were very supportive of each other and worked closely together, to some extent in-

Table 2. Continuity of care

	Know Your Midwife	Standard	Relative rate	99% CI
Fewer than 8 care givers seen during pregnancy	41/52 (79%)	24/49 (49%)	1.6	1.1– 2.4
Fewer than 3 midwives seen during labour	34/49* (69%)	22/46* (48%)	1.5	0.9– 2.3
Fewer than 3 doctors seen during labour	43/49* (88%)	35/46* (76%)	1.2	0.9– 1.5
Met intrapartum care giver during pregnancy	48/49* (98%)	9/46* (20%)	5.0	2.3–11.0

Data from 2 month casenotes study.
* Three women in each group either miscarried or delivered elsewhere.

Table 3. Women's view of the two systems of antenatal care

	Know Your Midwife	Standard	Relative rate	99% CI
Clinic waiting time <15 min*	169/275 (61%)	18/267 (7%)	9.1	5.0–16.6
Ability to discuss anxieties*	243/272 (89%)	200/261 (77%)	1.2	1.1– 1.3
Well prepared for labour*	144/275 (52%)	102/254 (40%)	1.3	1.0– 1.7
Enjoyment of labour*	104/246 (42%)	72/223 (32%)	1.3	1.0– 1.8
Feeling of control during labour*	103/246 (42%)	54/225 (24%)	1.7	1.2– 2.5
Satisfaction with pain relief*	121/209* (58%)	104/205* (51%)	1.1	0.9– 1.4
Well prepared for child care*	104/242 (43%)	64/222 (29%)	1.5	1.1– 2.1
Ability to discuss problems post-partum*	157/246 (64%)	112/220 (51%)	1.3	1.0– 1.5
Staff in labour 'very caring'*	252/275 (92%)	208/256 (81%)	1.1	1.0– 1.2

Date from * 37-week; * 2-day postnatal; and * 6-week postnatal questionnaires.
* Based on women who had normal deliveries.

Table 4. Maternal outcome

	Know Your Midwife	Standard	Relative rate	99% CI
Delivered during study	488	479		
Antenatal admission	123/484 (25%)	146/475 (31%)	0.8	0.6–1.1
Induction of labour*	51/465 (11%)	60/458 (13%)	0.8	0.5–1.3
Artificial rupture of membranes*	247/465 (53%)	270/454 (59%)	0.9	0.8–1.0
Augmentation of labour*	80/465 (17%)	114/458 (25%)	0.7	0.5–1.0
Length of first stage >6 hrs†	276/445 (62%)	229/439 (52%)	1.2	1.0–1.4
Epidural analgesia	88/479 (18%)	143/473 (30%)	0.6	0.4–0.8
Any analgesia other than Entonox	233/479 (49%)	293/473 (62%)	0.8	0.7–0.9
Operative vaginal delivery	56/479 (12%)	66/473 (14%)	0.8	0.5–1.3
Caesarean section	37/479 (8%)	35/473 (7%)	1.0	0.6–1.9
Episiotomy†	152/443 (34%)	185/438 (42%)	0.8	0.7–1.0
Vaginal tears†	184/443 (42%)	149/438 (34%)	1.2	1.0–1.5
Intact perineum†	107/443 (24%)	104/438 (24%)	1.0	0.7–1.4

* Elective caesareans excluded.
† All caesareans excluded.

dependently of other staff in the hospital. This led to some problems in the working relationship between 'Know Your Midwife' midwives and other personnel. All these difficulties should be taken into account when setting up similar schemes elsewhere.

It is not known how much of the observed effects in this study were due to enthusiasm, personality and efficiency of the midwives themselves rather than the scheme. There are still questions about whether the findings reported here are generalizable to a similar scheme worked by other midwives in other settings. Nevertheless, on the basis of the very encouraging findings we believe that this scheme, or a modification of it,

Table 5. Neonatal outcome

	Know Your Midwife	Standard	Relative rate	99% CI
Babies born during study*	478	471		
Birthweight <2500g	31/478 (6%)	38/471 (8%)	0.8	0.4–1.5
Apgar score				
<8 at one min	90/471 (19%)	91/467 (19%)	1.0	0.7–1.4
<8 at five min	17/470 (4%)	6/468 (1%)	2.8	0.8–9.5
Neonatal resuscitation	97/474 (20%)	128/465 (28%)	0.7	0.5–1.0
Admission to Special Care Nursery	23/475 (5%)	21/470 (4%)	1.1	0.5–2.3
Stillbirth or neonatal death	8/478 (2%)	4/471 (1%)	2.0	0.4–9.5

* 15 miscarriages and 3 terminations not included in this Table.

should be introduced widely elsewhere in such a way which allows further evaluation of its effects, particularly on neonatal outcome. The popularity of the scheme with women is no longer in question.

References

Association of Radical Midwives (1986). *The Vision – Proposals for the Future of the Maternity Services.* Ormskirk: ARM.

Chalmers, I., Hetherington, J., Newdick, M. et al. (1986). *The Oxford Database of Perinatal Trials: Developing a Register of Published Reports of Controlled Trials.* Controlled Clinical Trials 7: pp.306-324.

Flint, C. (1986). 'The Know Your Midwife Scheme'. *Midwife, Health Visitor and Community Nurse.* Vol.22, pp.168-169.

Maternity Services Advisory Committee (1982). 'Maternity care in action: Part 1 – antenatal care.' Crown Copyright, London.

Morris, J.A., Gardner,M.S. (1988). 'Calculating confidence intervals for relative risks (odds ratios) and standarized ratios and rates.' *British Medical Journal* 296: pp.1313-1316.

Slome, C.,Wetherbee, H., Daly, M., Christensen, K., Meglen, M., Theide, H. (1976). 'Effectiveness of certified nurse-midwives. A prospective evaluation study. *American Journal Obstetrics Gynaecology,* 124: pp.177-182.

Social Services Committee (1980). *Second Report on Perinatal and Neonatal Mortality.* HMSO, London.

Royal College of Midwives (1987). 'Report of the Royal College of Midwives on the role and education of the future midwife in the United Kingdom', Royal College of Midwives, London.

Royal College of Obstetricians and Gynaecologists (1982). 'Report of the RCOG working party on antenatal and intrapartum care.' Royal College of Obstetricians and Gynaecologists, London.

Runnerstrom, L. (1969). 'The effectiveness of nurse-midwifery in a supervised hospital environment.' *Bulletin of College of Nurse-Midwives* 14: pp.40-52.

Reproduced with kind permission from Midwifery, 5, 11-16, 1989.

A Dying Philosophy?

The debate continues:
Should midwives take a more active role in patient care?

In the July 1981 edition of the magazine 'Maternal and Child Health' Professor J. MacVicar who was Professor of Obstetrics of Leicester at the time, pointed out that 'there is an increasing number of mothers who come into an obstetric low risk category for themselves and their babies'. He went onto surmise that 'This may account for some of the decrease which has taken place in perinatal mortality'.[1]

In 1988 we are dealing with a population at less obstetric risk than has ever occurred in the whole history of womankind - women today are better educated, better nourished and better off than any generation of women have ever been, and most importantly of all, the babies they have are babies which they intend to have. No longer do women have 13 or 18 pregnancies because that is the lot of women - most women have no more than two or three pregnancies during their fertile years and they have those children because they want them. The babies who have always been (and still are) at most risk are the babies who come to the woman who has more than enough children already, the babies who come to women who are still children themselves at 13, 14 or 15.

Professor MacVicar also pointed out that nowadays 80 per cent of deliveries occur to women aged between 20 and 35 years the safest years for women to have babies.

It is bizarre that in an age when women are at the least risk obstetrically the caesarean rate is going up and up - from 4.3 per cent in 1970 to 11.3 per cent in 1987. And at the same time midwives who provide a service to women choosing to have home births, and especially those midwives who practise outside the National Health Service are at great risk of being hauled up before their Professional Conduct Machinery. I suggest that the two are not unrelated.

If most births are now occurring in low risk women their care can usefully be provided by the midwifery profession, with obstetricians dealing with the small number of women who have, or who develop, medical risks during pregnancy or labour. This has several benefits for the community at large, midwifery care is cheaper than obstetric care, not least because of the great discrepancy in the salaries of both professions, women who are enabled to get to know the midwives who will be delivering them need less antenatal admissions (cost saving) they feel more 'in control' of the situation during labour, they need less analgesia (another cost saving), they look back on their labour more favourably and they feel more prepared for motherhood.

A randomized controlled trial at St George's Hospital in Tooting between women cared for in the usual way and women cared for by a team of four midwives showed[2] that cost savings occurred in antenatal care because the women cared for by the midwives required less antenatal admissions, women cared for by the midwife team waited less time in the antenatal clinic which probably indicates cost savings for the community at large because employers were deprived of their employees for less time than those of working women in the Control Group.

The actual antenatal consultations cost less because women in the Midwife Group were seen by
• a receptionist
• a urine tester
• a weigher
• a doctor and
• someone chaperoning him - or if not actually chaperoning him, taking the woman's blood pressure for him.

All these staff cost money to employ. If they are all needed in order to provide the best antenatal care possible that is fine, but women in the Midwife Group much preferred their antenatal care, they found it easier to discuss anxieties, they looked back on their antenatal care more favourably and they saw less personnel during their pregnancy, and the personnel they met were the midwives who would be caring for them during labour - something that women have been requesting for many years.

Last year a booklet produced by the National Epidemiology Unit 'Where to be born - the debate and the evidence'[3] collated all research into place of birth during this century, they concluded that 'There is no evidence to support the claim that the safest policy is for all women to give birth in hospital' and 'There is some evidence, although not conclusive, that morbidity is higher amongst mothers and babies cared for in an institutional setting'. Their conclusions and growing evidence from GPs, [4, 5] statisticians like Marjorie Tew[6] (who for years has pointed out that the perinatal mortality rates would have fallen more quickly if women had been encouraged to give birth at home) are part of a rising chorus which claims that childbirth belongs to women and that the type of highly controlled and medicalized birth that most women are subjected to is inappropriate and not always in the best interests of women or their babies. As is seen in the area of caesarean section which is dependent on where the woman lives rather than on her obstetric profile (9.8 in Wessex compared with 12.8 per cent in Wales).

Not surprising then, that when this ageing philosophy 'that childbirth is only normal in retrospect' (as if the whole of life were any different), a philosophy which has such a profound effect on the controlling of women during a normal physiological function, is under attack, those who hold dear to such philosophy, whose very life's work has been the implementation of such a philosophy, attack back at those who represent most strongly the alternative to that philosophy 'Childbirth is a normal physiological function, women's bodies are beautifully and wondrously made and are designed to give birth, and when we interfere we interfere at our peril in a finely balanced process. Intervention should be used only when absolutely necessary and not as a first resort'. The group who represents this philosophy most strongly at the moment are the Independent Midwives who practise outside the National Health Service and deliver women at home, showing by their actions that women are able to give birth at home and midwives are able and appropriate to care for them - perhaps the present attack on them could be seen as the last throes of a dying philosophy.

References

1. MacVicar, J. (1981). 'Changing birth patterns during a period of declining births'. *Maternal and Child Health*, July.

2. Flint, C. (1988). 'Know Your Midwife' *Nursing Times*, Vol. 84, No 38. September 21.

3. Campbell, R., Macfarlane A. (1987). *Where to be born? The Debate and the Evidence.* National Perinatal Epidemiology Unit, Radcliffe Infirmary, Oxford.

4. Shearer, J. M. L. (1985). 'Five year prospective survey of risk of booking for a home birth in Essex.' *British Medical Journal*, Vol. 291, 23 November.

5. Damstra-Wijmenga S. M. I. (1984). 'Home confinement: the positive results in Holland.' *Journal of the Royal College of General Practitioners*, August.

6. Tew, M. (1985). 'Place of birth and perinatal mortality.' *Journal of the Royal College of General Practitioners*. August.

Reproduced with kind permission from Leicester Medical Review, Spring 1989

Riverside Midwife Teams

*A new maternity care scheme in Riverside gives women continuity of care
and reduces hospital costs*

For many years women have complained about the fragmentation of their care and the lack of carers during pregnancy, labour and the puerperium.

Micklethwaite, Beard and Shaw 1978[5]
'She would like, if it were possible, to have someone around her during labour who had given her some antenatal care.'

Short Report 1980[2]
'I think this is what women complain about most: they do not have continuity of care which they want very much during their antenatal visits but certainly during labour and delivery.'
'We recognize the difficulties of providing continuity of care throughout pregnancy and labour but consider that a measure of it can be obtained by better organization.'

MSAC 1982[4]
'Continuity of care. It is important that the woman should be able to build up a relationship of trust with the staff she meets, and efforts should be made to involve the same group of staff at each visit.'

RCOG 1982[7]
'It has been suggested to us that women should have the same midwife to attend them in labour as in the antenatal period. We consider this continuity of care to be an ideal aim and it may be possible in some circumstances.'

Parents Magazine 1986[6] (9,000 replies)
'Good communication between parents and the medical staff were helped where women saw the same doctor and midwife regularly...most mothers saw different people at almost every antenatal visit and were delivered by total strangers. While full of praise for the care they received, many women wished they could have had more continuity of care through pregnancy and beyond.'

Now, at last they are being listened to. The obstetricians and midwives of Riverside Health Authority from January 1989 are starting far-reaching changes in the way they deliver maternity care, which they see as the spearhead for future patterns of maternity care in the United Kingdom.

The new scheme
Under the new scheme most maternity care (except delivery) will take place either in, or near the woman's home. Once she has been and referred her pregnancy to her GP, the woman's next brush with the maternity services will be when she receives a letter detailing the team of six midwives who will care for her throughout her pregnancy, labour and puerperium. She will be given a photo of 'her' midwives and a date and a time when one of the midwives will visit her at home to take her obstetric history, a blood sample and plan the schedule of visits she will have during her pregnancy. Sometimes her antenatal consultation will be with the midwife team, sometimes with her GP and sometimes with the obstetric consultant, all depending on her needs and her level of risk.

The object is for her never to meet more than these eight health professionals plus the health visitor who will be working closely with the midwives during her pregnancy and labour. Indeed the midwives and health visitors will all be working in the same geographical patches since one of the aims of the scheme is to ensure an easier postnatal transfer to the health visitors and for the health visitors and midwives to work more closely together.

The woman will either be seen at home or at a local health clinic, where her obstetrician will also visit occasionally. Here she will also attend parentcraft classes and after the baby is born, mother and toddler groups, breast feeding clubs and nutritional meetings, such as 'Eating healthily on a budget' or 'Healthy eating without cooking', because the teams will be working closely with a dietician.

When the woman thinks she is in labour, having got to know the six midwives in her team during pregnancy, the woman will bleep the midwife team and whichever of the midwives is on call will answer the bleep. The usual practice will be for the midwife to visit the woman at home and assess the progress of the labour. Once it is appropriate for the woman to be transferred to hospital she and the midwife will set off with the partner, relatives and/or friends, probably by ambulance, but by car if available.

Once the midwife and the mother have arrived at the West London Hospital, the midwife will continue care - she has been writing the woman's notes (which the woman will have been carrying since the beginning of her pregnancy) - with referral to the medical staff if necessary.

The midwife will stay with the mother during labour and deliver the baby - the time needed should not be too great if she has judged the progress of labour well. According to the work of Klein[3], when women are assessed in early labour at home they spend less time in the delivery ward, have more normal deliveries and need less analgesia than women who spend most of their labour in the labour ward.

Once the baby has been delivered, preparations will be put in train for transfer home. The baby will be examined by the paediatrician on call and once all the necessary documentation has been carried out the new family and midwife will all transfer back home. Postnatal care will be given by the same team of midwives who, by now the mother will know very well. Obviously if the mother is unable to come home early she will stay in hospital, but she will be visited by 'her' midwives while she is on the postnatal ward.

The benefits

It is thought that the benefits for women will be that they will enjoy being able to get to know their midwives. Their reactions are being assessed with the use of the Edinburgh Postnatal Depression Score at approximately six weeks following delivery and the results will be compared with those obtained from women prior to the start of the scheme.

The midwives' job satisfaction levels are being assessed with a questionnaire which was given out to all midwives prior to the inception of the scheme. This will be distributed again once the scheme has been in operation for about nine months to see if there are any changes in attitudes of the midwives. It is interesting that although no advertisements have yet been put out for midwife team members, every post brings letters from midwives all over the United Kingdom applying for a position in one of the teams. The midwives, it seems, can hardly contain themselves in their eagerness to start working in this way.

An example of one off duty is shown in Figure 1. The off duty will be planned for a year in advance and there will nearly always be a member of the team on holiday so that usually there will be five midwives working at any time; the midwives will aim to book six new women each week, to deliver six women each week and give postnatal care for the six women who deliver each week.

	M	T	W	Th	F	S	S	M	T	W	Th	F	S	S	M	T	W	Th	F	S	S	M	T	W	Th	F	S	S	M	T	W	Th	F	S	S
1	L	D	D	1	2	1	E2	E	1	2	E	E	D	D	L	D	D	E	1	E2	1	2	E	1	2	E	D	D	1	2	E	E	E	D	D
2	L	D	D	E	1	E2	1	2	E	1	2	E	D	D	1	2	E	E	E	D	D	L	D	D	1	2	1	E2	E	1	2	E	E	D	D
3	1	2	E	E	E	D	D	L	D	D	1	2	1	E2	E	1	2	E	E	D	D	L	D	D	E	1	E2	1	2	E	1	2	E	D	D
4	E	1	2	E	E	D	D	L	D	D	E	1	E2	1	2	E	1	2	E	D	D	1	2	E	E	E	D	D	L	D	D	1	2	1	E2
5	2	E	1	2	E	D	D	1	2	E	E	E	D	D	L	D	D	1	2	1	E2	E	1	2	E	E	D	D	L	D	D	E	1	E2	1
6	COVER FOR ANNUAL LEAVE, REFRESHER COURSE, OVERTIME, SICK LEAVE																																		

Fig. 1

Many GPs are enthusiastic about the teams since they are looking forward to working more closely with midwives. They will be able to contact them at any time (as can the women) and they will be assured that they will be speaking to a midwife they know. They feel that communications will be much better under the new scheme.

The obstetrician who will be medically supporting the team, Mr Roger Marwood, is happy to be working closely with his midwife colleagues; he sees the teams as providing a more intimate experience for women within the safety of the present hospital set up.

This new scheme is the brain child of the Director of Midwifery Services, Suzanne Truttero. She is anxious to see midwives practising their role fully for the benefit of both women and the midwifery profession.

The Health Authority is also happy to see women occupying maternity beds for shorter lengths of time than previously, because this could enable great cost savings to be made. The Health Authority has recently rationalized its maternity services and this scheme fits in well with its basic philosophy to decentralise and improve the quality of care, and at the same time become more cost effective. Previous research has shown that women cared for in this way seem to need less antenatal admissions and less analgesia.[1]

The health visitors are also looking forward to working more closely with their midwife colleagues. Most of them feel that what is happening today in Riverside, will tomorrow be the norm for all pregnant women.

The philosophy underlying Riverside's approach is that all women are entitled to be cared for by health professionals they have been able to get to know during their pregnancy and that it is iniquitous that so many women are cared for by strangers during one of their most intimate experiences.

References

1. Flint, C., Poulengeris, P. (1987). 'The Know Your Midwife Report.' Pub 49 Peckarmans Wood. London .
2. HMSO. (1980). *Second Report from the Social Services Committee. Session (1979-80), Perinatal and Neonatal Mortality*. 19th June.HMSO.
3. Klein, M., Lloyd, I., Redman C., Bull, M., Turnbull, A. C. (1983). 'A comparison of low-risk women booked for delivery in two different systems of care.' *British Journal of Obstetrics and Gynaecology*. 90, pp.118-28.
4. Maternity Services Advisory Committee (1982). 'Maternity care in action. Part 1 - Antenatal Care.' Crown Copyright.
5. Micklethwaite, Lady P., Beard, Professor R., Shaw, Kathleen (1978). 'Expectations of a pregnant woman in relation to her treatment.' *British Medical Journal*. 2, pp.188-191.
6. Parents Magazine (1986). 'BIRTH - 9000 mothers speak out. Birth Survey 1986 - results.' No 128 November.
7. Royal College of Obstetricians and Gynaecologists (1982). 'Report of the RCOG working party on antenatal and intrapartum care.'

Reproduced with kind permission from Midwife, Health Visitor and Community Nurse, Vol. 25, No. 3, March 1989.

To My Dear Sisters in New Zealand

Midwifery Consultant to Riverside Health Authority and Independent Midwife, Caroline is wife and mother to three adult children. Author of 'Sensitive Midwifery' and co-author of 'Community Midwifery'

Until the day I die one of the great highlights of my life will always be the wonderful week I spent with the midwives of New Zealand in August 1988 - a time when I was acutely conscious of history being made and brave decisions being taken. The time when the midwives of New Zealand decided to form their own College of Midwives and break from the Nurses Association. A frightening decision, one surrounded by doubts and a wish to be able to see into the future to check out that it was the right decision and not one taken in a moment of madness and impulse. The siren call 'stay with us we are so much bigger and therefore so much more influential' sounds SO reasonable but did size ever win anything?. I doubt it.

Women at this time probably more than at any other in the whole history of womankind need midwives more than ever before. Why am I suggesting this? I am suggesting this because women in 1989 are at a lower obstetric risk than they have ever been and yet they are being subjected to greater and greater levels of intervention.

Professor J. MacVicar, Professor of Obstetrics at Leicester (UK) pointed out in an article in *Maternal and Child Health* that 'there is an increasing number of mothers who come into an obstetric low risk category for themselves and their babies'. He went on to surmise that 'this may account for some of the decrease which has taken place in perinatal mortality'.

The reason that women are in such a favourable state for giving birth is that women today are better educated, better nourished and better off than any generation of women have ever been and most importantly of all, the babies they have are babies which they intend to have. Women in 1989 do not have 13 or 18 pregnancies just because that is the lot of women - most women have no more than 2 or 3 pregnancies during their fertile years and they have those children because they want them. The babies who have always been at the most risk are the babies who come to the woman who has more than enough children already or the babies who come to women who are still children themselves at 13, 14 or 15.

Nowadays 80 per cent of deliveries occur to women aged between 20 and 35 years - the safest years for women to have babies and yet the Caesarean section rate is going up, in the UK from 4.3 per cent in 1970 to 11.3 per cent in 1987, and the whole concept of birth as a normal or even POSSIBLE event seems to be fading. Every women you meet has either 'needed' an episiotomy because the baby was 'in distress' or 'needed' forceps because the mother was exhausted or 'needed' a fetal scalp electrode because the baby was 'in distress', or has had a doctor who 'saved my life' or who 'saved the baby's life'. The concept of birth as being something which women are designed to do and whose bodies are wondrously and beautifully made to do is being lost. As birth is taken out of homes and into hospitals which become more and more cluttered with the panoply of equipment which bleeps, flashes, or computes, midwives tend to become 'nurses' tending these poor invalids who are 'at risk' and whose babies are in peril.

Only by staying separate, only by standing strong can midwives hope to protect women from the seductive onslaught of pathological childbirth, 'we're only doing it for the baby's sake, my dear'.

Eventually the madness of this situation will percolate into the mass consciousness - at a time when economics are important and ways of providing cost effective health care are being sought, the realization that midwifery care is not only effective but also cheaper will win us through. Our care is cheaper and more cost effective, not just because of the great discrepancy in the salaries of both professions. Women who are able to get to know the midwives who will be delivering them need less antenatal admissions (cost saving), they feel more 'in control' of the situation during labour, they need less analgesia (another cost saving), they look back on labour more favourably and they feel more prepared for motherhood.

Women looked after by the 'Know Your Midwife' team waited less time at the antenatal clinic which probably indicates cost savings for the community at large because employers were deprived of their employees for less time than those of working women in the Control Group. Midwives use the technological aids available for birth, but they use them rationally and appear to be able to look at every woman as an individual with individual needs and not to treat ALL WOMEN with specific equipment because IT'S ROUTINE. If anything is done as a 'routine' in childbirth it needs to be looked at and challenged - it may be entirely appropriate for many women but in something so unique as birth it cannot be right for all women regardless.

In 1987 a booklet produced by the National Epidemiology Unit 'Where to be Born - the debate and the evidence' collated all research on the place of birth during this century. They concluded that 'there is no evidence to support the claim that the safest policy is for all women to give birth in hospital' and 'there is some evidence, although not conclusive, that morbidity is higher among mothers and babies cared for in an institutional setting'. Their conclusions and growing evidence from GP's and statisticians like Majorie Tew who for years has pointed out that the perinatal mortality rates would have fallen more quickly if women had been encouraged to give birth at home are part of a rising chorus which claims that childbirth belongs to women and that the type of highly controlled and medicalized birth that many women are subjected to is inappropriate and not always in the best interests of women or their babies.

The women of New Zealand need strong, identifiable midwives - don't fret because there are so few of you - if just one person can change and influence the world, there's more than enough of you – dear midwives.

References

MacVicar, J. (1981). 'Changing birth patterns during a period of declining births.' *Maternal and Child Health*, July .

Flint, C. (1988). 'Know Your Midwife' *Nursing Times* September 21, Vol 84, No. 38

Campbell, R., MacFarlene A. (1987). *Where to be born? The Debate and the evidence* National Perinatal Epidemiology Unit, Radcliffe Infirmary, Oxford.

Shearer, J.M.L. (1985). 'Five Year Prospective survey of risk of booking for a home birth in Essex.' *British Medical Journal*, Vol. 291, 23 December .

Damstra-Wijmenga S.M.I. (1984). 'Home confinement: the positive results in Holland.' *Journal of the Royal College of General Practitioners*, August.

Tew, M., (1985). 'Place of birth and perinatal mortality.' *Journal of the Royal College of General Practitioners*, August.

Reproduced with kind permission from Journal of the New Zealand College of Midwives, September 1989.

Antenatal Care in the Future

Women's complaints about their antenatal care have remained constant over the past two decades. They object to waiting for long periods of time to be seen by someone they don't know for a cursory consultation. Cartwright (1979) and Arnold (1984) showed that antenatal care is aimed inappropriately - women at high risk (who may not be very clean or who don't speak English) are often relegated to the most junior doctor or midwife for their consultation, while women at low risk (middle class, well nourished and well educated: the solicitors' accountants and doctors' wives) are frequently given a gold star or other emblem on their notes. They are seen by the consultant and are destined to be on the receiving end of overmedicalized birth technologies, with too many inductions of labour, instrumental deliveries and an overuse of epidurals.

Hall et al (1980) pointed out that the schedule to which we religiously adhere for antenatal consultations, i.e. every month until 28 weeks, then every fortnight until 36 weeks and after that every week, has no basis in either fact, researched benefits or usefulness. The Royal College of Obstetricians and Gynaecologists recommended Hall et als. schedule as long ago as 1982, but remarkably few institutions have taken up these suggestions.

Shared care with the GP has been seen as a more efficient way of palming off the less interesting cases at the same time as cutting down women's need to travel to the hospital. Each hospital and each consultant obstetrician varies the number of times women having shared care have to return to the hospital. Often these are at the times when something important may happen or is happening, such as at 28 weeks when the onset of pre-eclampsia may be detected and blood samples have to be taken.

Many obstetricians have a selection of favoured GP's who are allowed to carry out the whole of the antenatal care procedure. Sometimes these GP's are favoured because they have exhibited specific obstetric skills in the past, but the relationship may be a purely social one.

Effective Care in Pregnancy and Childbirth (Chalmers et al, 1989), is a collation of almost all randomized controlled trials pertaining to effective care in childbirth. Since it was published and became available to the media and to vocal pressure groups, many obstetricians are beginning to realize that their days as the providers of maternity care to all women are numbered. Basically the type of highly medicalized, often anxiety-provoking care that they often provide is inappropriate to most women. The most forward-looking obstetricians are beginning to look at ways of damage limitation and at where to direct antenatal care in the future.

GP's have for many years been carrying out shared care but there has been little research into its effectiveness. In a study of 577 women receiving shared care from their GP's (Flint and Poulengeris, 1987) women enjoyed their antenatal care from their GP's. This was because they did not have to wait very long to be seen and GP's were more helpful with anxieties than their hospital counterparts (but the research shows that no doctors were as helpful as midwives).

However, it was apparent that although women had enjoyed their antenatal care from their GP's they suffered as a result during labour. They felt less prepared, their perception of how well they had managed were lower and their feelings of being in control were significantly lower than those of a group having full hospital care and a group being looked after by four midwives whom they were able to get to know during pregnancy and who were with them during labour.

It has been well documented for many years that women's greatest desire is to have with them during labour someone they already know and have received care from. This is not an unusual concept - to have someone familiar during the most intimate experience in life would seem to be eminently sensible. The converse would seem the bizarre alternative rather than the norm as it is now.

My hope for the future of antenatal care is simple. I see pregnancy as the precursor to the most responsible role any human being takes on - that of becoming a parent. Women want care providers who are prepared to accompany them on a path that starts with pregnancy diagnosis and ends with a thriving baby. If we are not prepared to provide that continuum because our own needs are too great, we have too many other irons in the fire, or we lack the imagination to see how important this is to women, then I suggest that we should not be offering fragmented parts of the care.

GP care during pregnancy is often good, but most GPs abandon women when they need a familiar face most intensely, i.e. during labour. Obstetricians concentrate on processing as many women as possible that is usually helpful neither to the obstetrician nor to the client. Midwives are available at all stages of the childbirth continuum but often proffer excuses as to why continuity of care can't be provided - usually because it needs a degree of flexibility and imagination that takes great effort. This is a difficult problem, but not unsolvable, as has been shown in several areas. It is time those of us who provide care for pregnant women began listening to their needs and providing for them. We might find it mutually beneficial.

References

Arnold, M. (1984). *The Tricycle of Deprivation.* M A Thesis.

Cartwright, A. (1979). *The Dignity of Labour?* Tavistock, London.

Chalmers, I., Enkin, M.W., Keirse, M.J.N.C (1989). *Effective Care in Pregnancy and Childbirth*, Oxford: Oxford University Press.

Flint, C., Poulengeris, P. (1987). *The Know Your Midwife Report,* MIDIRS, Bristol.

Hall, M.H., Ching, P.K., MacGillivray, I. (1980). Is routine antenatal care worthwhile? *Lancet* ii: pp.78-80.

Royal College of Obstetricians and Gynaecologists (1982). *Report of the RCOG working Party on Antenatal and Intrapartum Care.*

Reproduced with kind permission from British Journal of Hospital Medicine, Vol 47/2, 1992

Name, Set and Match

Better maternity care is possible if pregnant women are given a named midwife, says Caroline Flint

The recent report from the House of Commons health committee on maternity services recommends midwives should have their own caseloads and every woman should be able to get to know a midwife during the antenatal period who would be with her in labour and deliver the baby.

Recently, two conferences were held by the Nuffield Institute to address the problem, and to discuss a working document called '*Who's Left Holding the Baby?*', which detailed the costs and how the named midwife concept could be achieved. The *Patient's Charter* group also issued a document called *The Named Midwife* which discusses how the concept would work. This has been sent to all midwives.

In the UK, there are more than 100,000 qualified midwives, but only 34,000 are actually registered as practising. This in itself is an extraordinary phenomenon: that midwives who have spent a long time training and qualifying do not go on to do the job for which they trained although there is considerable personal investment of time, energy and effort. This large drop-out rate may indicate a lack of satisfaction with the job as it is carried out in the NHS.

In *Who's Left Holding the Baby?* one problem identified in modern maternity care is that midwives are seen as people who staff a place such as an antenatal clinic, antenatal ward, labour ward or the community, when what women really need is for the midwife to be where they are, when they need her. Sometimes this is in their homes, and sometimes in the hospital. If we move away from the concept of staffing places or areas to the concept of staffing women, levels of staff might conceivably be changed and be much more flexible.

Who's Left Holding the Baby? suggests that if every midwife were to take on a caseload of between 24 and 38 women a year, women would be able to have a named midwife and would probably have happier childbirth experiences.

It is expected that each midwife who takes on, say, 36 women would work with another midwife so each would have a caseload of 36 women and one of them would be available when the other was not. These midwives would probably be on call all the time they were not working but, as they would not be called more than once a week, this would be less arduous than it sounds.

At the moment midwives work more than 37 hours a week, which is equivalent to 1,687 hours per midwife each year. As these hours would be worked more intensely during working times, the midwives could take three months' holiday. So if we had two midwives, called Janet and Mary, Janet could decide to take her holidays during March, July and November, and Mary could decide to take her holidays during January, May and September. Each of them would take on 36 women due to deliver in the intervening months (see above).

They would work out between them when they were going to have their holidays, and if there were a particular month which always seemed to have a lot of babies, then neither would take a holiday during that month.

If we view the scene in April it is easy to see how it would work. The women who are due in November and December are not yet 12 weeks' pregnant, and would probably not have booked with these midwives. The women who are due in January, February and March would more or less have delivered and finished their postnatal care. So Janet would have 24 women to look after and Mary would have 20. Janet is looking forward to a month's holiday in July while Mary has a month's holiday in May and another in September.

To provide full care for 24 women is not difficult. Each woman could be given the normal type of antenatal care so that she was seen regularly by her midwife throughout her pregnancy. Each woman could also see her GP or an obstetrician for an agreed number of visits, but she would be secure in the knowledge that she had a named midwife, who would carry a long-range pager so that 'her' women had access to her.

On going into labour a woman would bleep her midwife, who would go to her home and assess the progress of labour. When appropriate, the midwife would accompany the women to hospital to deliver her baby, or deliver her at home. Assessing women at home would eliminate what have been called 'category X' patients, estimated to be between 30 and 40 per cent of any labour ward's admissions and who cost hospitals up to £29,000 per month. These are women who go to the labour ward to be assessed, but who are not in established labour and who are either sent home again or sent to the antenatal ward overnight, where they often have labour induced just because they are there. Inducing a labour which is not physiologically ready to start often leads to greater intervention at delivery, such as a caesarean section or forceps delivery, and has cost implications.

With the system described here, women could deliver their babies at home or in hospital, whether they were low or high obstetric risks. Their need for obstetric input could be catered for in a flexible system in which their named midwife was with them when they needed her.

References

Nuffield Institute for Health Service Studies. (1992). *Who's Left Holding the Baby? An Organizational Framework for Making the Most of the Maternity Service.* The Nuffield Institute for Health Services Studies.

The Patient's Charter Group. (1992). *The Named Midwife.* London.

Ball, J. (1992). *Birthrate, Using clinical indicators to access case-mix, workload outcomes and staffing needs in intrapartum care and for predicting postnatal beds needs.* The Nuffield Institute for Health Service Studies.

Reproduced with kind permission from Health Service Journal, 23 July 1992.

Hailing a New Philosophy

Implementing the recommendations contained in the 'Changing Childbirth' report means midwives will have to adopt a revolutionary new way of working. But Caroline Flint believes they have the skills necessary to meet the challenge

The fundamental principle underpinning all the proposals outlined in the document *Changing Childbirth*[1] is that women should be in control of their birth giving: that they should have choice and continuity of care.

Women are thus able to take responsibility for birth giving, and the health professionals involved should enable this to happen. At the same time, health professionals, especially midwives, should take responsibility for their own practice.

Basic to the underlying philosophy of the document is the statement 'The woman and her baby should be at the centre of all planning and provision of maternity care.' This does not sound like a revolutionary statement. After all, who is maternity care provided for but mothers and their babies? But do not be deceived. This fundamental principle actually means a complete change in the way that maternity care will be provided in future.

During the past two decades, childbirth has been seen as a hazardous and dangerous process through which a woman and her baby must travel before entering the new world of parenthood. The woman's body has been perceived as harmful and hazardous to her baby, and the underlying principle of maternity care has been to get the baby out of the woman's body as quickly as possible. To this end, the woman's body has been controlled and contained, her contractions have been speeded up or slowed down, and the baby has been delivered as opposed to the woman giving birth to her child.

This has not, of course, happened to all women. In almost every labour ward in the country, however, there has been the perception that a high risk process is taking place and an atmosphere of barely disguised panic has ensured.

Change in emphasis

Changing Childbirth and its precursor[1] hail a completely new philosophy for childbearing women. It is that 'a woman gives birth, that the pregnancy is her pregnancy, the labour is her labour, the birth is her birth and the baby is her baby. The child belongs to the woman and her partner, not anybody else. The process should not be controlled or in any interfered with without real medical necessity, and the woman's express desire and agreement. What differences can this enormous change in emphasis bring?

For women, it will bring awareness, probably even sooner than usual, that the responsibility for this human being is her own and that however difficult, demanding or cranky the baby happens to be, it is her baby and her responsibility.

This awareness, the realization that for the rest of her life this unique individual is part of her, can weigh heavily at first: until recently it seems to have been softened unrealistically by hospital staff taking on the responsibility. The other side of the acceptance of greater responsibility is the likelihood of increased confidence when a woman embarks on motherhood. The person who has made all the decisions, who has felt in control, appears to feel more confident than the woman who has been organized and controlled.

This single factor is of enormous importance. It is often the mother who provides the early and most basic teaching of her child, who counts and names objects and reads *Thomas the Tank Engine* and *Postman Pat* . It is often also she who chooses the first school, enables her child to get there and collects the insides of kitchen rolls for projects. How much more easily does all this come to her if she has been in control of her pregnancy and labour?

And what changes does the new philosophy of *Changing Childbirth* represent for the midwife? Again, probably the taking on of greater responsibility. It goes without saying that midwives must listen to women. Midwives must listen when they say: 'I want to know the midwife who looks after me all through my pregnancy and is with me during labour'. *Changing Childbirth* is the second government report to underline this important need. And how will midwives comply with this request? A few probably will continue as they do now, working shifts in hospitals, but it is likely that they will be providing cover for the labour and postnatal wards. It is also likely that most midwives will be working in a manner that is far more like that of the independent midwives – taking on their own caseloads.

Tentative figures suggest that each full time midwife will need to take on between 35 and 40 women a year [3], providing all their pregnancy, labour and postnatal care. Midwives will probably find it easier to work in partnership with other midwives, but their caseload of women will be just that – their caseload. Most midwives will deliver all these women, being on-call for them and responsive to their needs.

As a midwife who has been on-call for the past 12 years, I can report that it is not as bad as it sounds. In fact, once maternity care becomes part of your life you fit it around everything else. So I often go to the theatre, to concerts and out for meals in restaurants. I see my adult children frequently, have friends and relatives to stay and entertain regularly.

Modern communication systems make it possible for midwives to go wherever they need or want and still be accessible to the women they are caring for. Are they always ringing or bleeping? The answer is no. If a woman knows she is to see the midwife on Tuesday, she rarely calls in between. If these women know that can speak to the midwife whenever they want, they feel relaxed and so do not call often. If a midwife takes on a caseload of 36 women annually, she can have three month's holiday a year. This means working the same number of hours as she currently does, but they would be organized differently and fitted into life in a way that shift work makes impossible.

Three month's holiday
The Royal College of Midwives has worked hard to secure a 37.5 hour week for the profession, and it is an enormous benefit, but within that rather inflexible time span it can be impossible to provide total care.

But when working hours are calculated annually, with seven weeks' holiday included, we are looking at 1,687.5 hours per midwife. If each woman takes approximately 45 hours of midwife time (seven- and- a-half antenatal, 16 labour care, 14 postnatal and seven-and-a-half administration and travelling), 36 women will require 1,620 hours and 37 need 1,665 hours.

Anything above a caseload of 37 women would take too many hours for one midwife on her own, but would be feasible if some of the antenatal care was provided by the GP or obstetrician, or if the recommendations of the Royal College of Obstetricians for fewer antenatal visits were adopted. Each area will need to work out its preferred route. With such a system it does not matter where the woman decides to deliver or whether she is high or low risk, her midwife will always be there for her. If she is delivering in hospital it is likely that the midwife will transfer her from home during the labour and will return her there after the delivery.

If the woman is at very high risk, the start of labour may also take place in hospital. If a Caesarean section is needed, the woman's midwife will be beside her, caring for the baby and helping to get breastfeeding started right away.

A new way of working will require a new attitude among midwives. But the skills are already there, it just takes a change in emphasis. Instead of staffing physical spaces – the antenatal clinic, the community, the postnatal ward – midwives will need to staff women.

References
1. Department of Health (1993). *Changing Childbirth*. Report of the Expert Maternity Group. London: HMSO.
2. House of Commons Select Committee on Health (1992). *Second Report on Maternity Services*. London: HMSO.
3. Ball, J. et al.(1992). *Who's left holding the baby? An organizational framework for making the most of midwifery services*. London: The Nuffield Institute for Health Services.

Reproduced with kind permission from Nursing Standard ,Vol. 8, No. 20, 19 February 1994

Books for Midwives Press

Books for Midwives Press, in joint collaboration with the Royal College of Midwives, publish books written by experts in the midwifery field to meet the practical needs of the working midwife and midwifery student. Below is a list of our current and forthcoming titles:

Current titles

A Short History of Clinical Midwifery	Philip Rhodes	£17.95
Super-Vision	ARM	£9.95
Teaching Physical Skill for the Childbearing Year	Eileen Brayshaw & Pauline Wright	£10.95
HIV Infection in Pregnancy	Caroline Shepherd	£6.95
Antenatal Investigations	Maureen Boyle	£6.95
Understanding Obstetric Ultrasound	Jean Proud	£10.95
MIRIAD	NPEU	£14.95
Aquanatal Exercises	Gillian Hawksworth	£6.95
Holding On?	Hazel McHaffie	£9.95
Reactions to Motherhood	Jean Ball	£10.95
Sexuality and Motherhood	Irene Walton	£10.95
Legal Aspects of Midwifery	Bridgit Dimond	£12.95
Midwives and 'Changing Childbirth'	Walton & Hamilton	£9.95
Waterbirth	Dianne Garland	£10.95
The Pregnant Drug Addict	Catherine Siney	£9.95

If you would like to receive details about future titles and be placed on our mailing list, please send your details to the address given below.

Please order *Books for Midwives Press* titles from your usual bookseller and encourage them to stock midwifery titles. If you prefer you can order from us by sending a cheque (made payable to *Books for Midwives Press*) to the address below or by telephoning 0161-929-0929 for credit/debit card orders (Access/Visa/Switch/Delta). For overseas postage please add 25% of total price. All UK orders are sent postage free.

Please send orders or requests for catalogues/information to:

BOOKS FOR MIDWIVES PRESS
Freepost WA1836
Hale
Cheshire
WA15 9BR
0161 929 0929